Communicating with Dying People and their Relatives

Jean Lugton

Foreword by
Dorothy Whyte

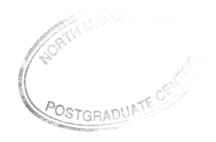
Radcliffe Medical Press

GNWC

(EN062)

Radcliffe Medical Press Ltd
18 Marcham Road
Abingdon
Oxon OX14 1AA
United Kingdom

www.radcliffe-oxford.com
The Radcliffe Medical Press electronic catalogue and online ordering facility.
Direct sales to anywhere in the world.

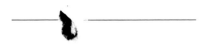

© 2002 Jean Lugton

Reprinted 2002

British Library Cataloguing in Publication Data

A catalogue record for this book is available from the British Library.

ISBN 1 85775 584 7

Typeset by Acorn Bookwork, Salisbury, Wiltshire
Printed and bound by TJ International Ltd., Padstow, Cornwall

Contents

Foreword

Having been aware of Jean Lugton's work in breast cancer and on communication in terminal care, I was delighted to have a preview of this book. As I read through it, I was increasingly impressed by the way in which research and theory have been woven together in a way that makes sense for practice.

Much has been written and learned about communicating with dying people but it is evident that practice in some areas has changed very little. In this book, Jean Lugton expounds the principles of making communication more effective, making reference to her own clinical practice, relevant literature and research. The inclusion of interview extracts from her original research gives life and substance to the theoretical concepts discussed. The fact that some of these extracts describe relationships with nurses that patients or relatives found supportive is both satisfying and encouraging. It seems that we are making progress on some fronts!

While the focus of the book is very much on nursing, the importance of nurses contributing effectively to multiprofessional teamwork is stressed. In today's healthcare system, as it attempts to meet the needs of an increasingly informed public, the need for understanding of, and respect for, each other's roles has never been greater. We need to be able to move on from protecting our professional boundaries to believing that there is enough need out there to keep us all fully occupied. We can then focus without distraction on the needs of patients and families facing the threats and challenges of the palliative care experience. It does not detract from this primary aim to plan in support for the professionals engaged with patients and families on their journey. This book makes an important contribution to the consideration of these issues.

One of the pleasures for me was the discussion of support for the family. This is not seen as a luxury for which there may not be sufficient time, but as an essential part of caring for people requiring palliative care. The way in which professionals may help family members to communicate with each other when painful issues and uncertainties raise barriers between them is very helpfully described. The sensitivity which must be exercised in this delicate area is also acknowledged. The importance for many people, living through such stressful experiences, of having a confidante outside the family system underlines the importance of skilled and empathic nursing support. Jean Lugton has the honesty to acknowledge that though we know the value of openness and the strength it can give, we must also accept the right of individuals to keep their own counsel if this is their conscious decision. This perhaps demonstrates the breadth and depth of this book, in which the reader can sense that while the writer has a wealth of academic knowledge on which to draw, the realities and dilemmas of nursing practice are very much to the foreground of her thinking.

The style of the book is very readable and the questions at the end of each chapter encourage reflection and discussion.

It is a book that will be welcomed by students, teachers and practitioners.

Dorothy Whyte BA PhD RSCN RGN HV RNT
Honorary Fellow
Department of Nursing Studies
University of Edinburgh
October 2001

About the author

Jean Lugton PhD MA (Hons) MSc SRN RNT is a Health Visitor and External Examiner for the Specialist Practitioner Course in Palliative Care at Dundee University. She trained as a nurse in Liverpool, where she was a ward sister for four years before qualifying as a nurse teacher in Edinburgh, and taking her sociology honours degree. She worked as a nurse teacher in North Lothian College whilst completing her MSc thesis. Then, when Education Officer at St Columba's Hospice in Edinburgh, she developed the first courses in palliative nursing in Scotland and undertook a research study exploring the support needs of relatives of Hospice patients. The Hospice now offers a degree course in Nursing Studies: Palliative Care. Later, as a Macmillan Research Fellow, she undertook her PhD, exploring the complementary roles of professional and informal support for patients with breast cancer. Recently, following an invitation from nursing bodies in Japan she has lectured there on palliative care.

1

Terminal illness

A terminal illness may be defined as one for which no cure is available and which will bring about the death of the person in the fairly near future. However, it is not always easy to recognise when the terminal phase of an illness has been reached. Our care of the dying begins at the time of the fatal diagnosis and not just within the last weeks or days of life.

Patients and their relatives need support and counselling to enable them to cope with the shattering impact of the diagnosis, whether they are asked to face it immediately, or whether it comes as a slowly dawning realisation. It is, therefore, more helpful to speak about 'palliative care' than 'terminal care'.

Palliative care implies actively endeavouring to relieve physical, psychosocial, and spiritual distress and presents great challenges to the carers in the difficult areas of treatment and communication.

Quality of life, not quantity, becomes the aim of care. Knowledge of how people relate to their experience of illness is more important than information about the particular disease which will cause them to die. People can be encouraged to live 'actively' until their last days rather than becoming depressed and resigned to their fate. When a terminal illness has been diagnosed, there may be a temptation by nurses and relatives to overprotect the person, thus preventing him or her from leading as full a life as possible.

Importance of good communication in palliative care

Research has shown that patients with cancer who receive psychological support experience a greater sense of well being and may even survive for longer (Fallowfield 1995). However, support previously available in the form of cohesive family structures or organised religion has decreased. Also, increasingly, patients with cancer will require support while living with the disease, often having complex therapies over months or even years. In some hospitals, cancer caring centres have been set up to help people with cancer to find answers to questions they may have:

- How am I going to deal with this?
- What questions should I have asked the doctor but didn't?
- Who am I going to turn to?
- I will be having medical treatment but is there anything else I can do to make myself feel better?

At the centres, there are usually trained therapists, including a psychologist, clinical nurse specialist and complementary therapies specialists to facilitate group support and families' and friends' support (Jencks 1995). The Expert Advisory Group on Cancer (Calman and Hine 1995) advocated a reorganisation of cancer services to bring about 'seamless care' between secondary and primary care. Reorganisation within primary care is still in its early stages. In a small study, exploring access to community services by people with a terminal illness, Beaver *et al.* (2000) found that lay carers did not always receive the information and support they needed. Ineffective communication between patients, lay carers and primary healthcare teams, caused confusion. Different health-care professionals recommended different care packages. Lay carers often did not know in advance if they were going to receive assistance, for example, night sitting services. Beaver *et al.* (2000) concluded that:

> '*The findings of this study indicate that users would welcome more effective communication between different professionals in planning a package of care.*'

Another small study by Adam (2000) explored how well carers perceived they were prepared by hospital staff to care for terminally ill relatives at home. She found that factors that influenced coping were the patients' acceptance of them as carers and the preparation and support patients and carers received from health professionals, family and friends. Most carers were satisfied with the information they received about the patient's diagnosis and prognosis but many would have welcomed more information about medication.

As a result of my research with patients with breast cancer (Lugton 1997), a service was set up with health visitors acting as resource personnel for colleagues and liaising with a hospital breast cancer unit. The health visitors underwent a short education programme to increase their ability to help patients in several key areas. All the health visitors described the support of patients in the community with treated breast cancer as important. While they felt that their support to patients was mainly psychological, they also described giving medical information and assisting with a number of social problems.

Maintaining hope

In palliative care, where patients have to live with a degree of uncertainty as to the possible course their illness may take and the length of life they may expect, hope is a major issue. People's emotional responses to terminal illness can determine whether they live actively and positively, maintaining a hopeful outlook, or whether they are consumed by fear of what is happening to them or have anxieties about the future. A terminal illness is often described as a 'hopeless' situation, yet despairing attitudes about the effectiveness of treatment or about the person's ability to respond to the knowledge of impending death may mean that avenues for the relief of distressing symptoms are not fully explored, or that communications with the family or with healthcare professionals are blocked. It is important to maintain the delicate balance between realistic hope and acceptance of the inevitable in palliative care. Dying people and their relatives need encouragement to believe that symptoms can be controlled or alleviated even when the disease is incurable, that dignity can be maintained and that they themselves will have the courage as well as support from professionals to enable them to cope with a crisis.

This can only be achieved in an atmosphere of honesty and trust between patients, relatives and professionals. When people are given misleading information, or when information is withheld from them, they often reach their own conclusions about the true state of affairs from what their bodies are telling them and from their reflections on what has not been said. Paradoxically, total truth may not be very helpful either, since emphasising only the terminal nature of the illness and not the treatment and care that are still available may drive dying people and their relatives to complete despair.

Patients are now being told their diagnosis earlier and in greater detail than before. The alleviation of physical distress does not depend exclusively on giving skilled physical care. It also depends on understanding and helping dying people with their fears. It is inevitable that patients and relatives will experience varying degrees of anxiety at the time a terminal illness is diagnosed, when there are signs of recurrence, or when it appears that a terminal phase has been reached. Slevin *et al.* (1990) found that patients continue to opt for radical treatment even where there is minimal chance of benefit.

Our attitudes and actions can create a climate of hope for patients. Herth (1990) found that having one's individuality respected helped to facilitate hope. Kreiger (1982) described four phases of a terminal illness and the hopes the patient may have during each of these phases.

1 In the first phase, the patient hopes that there has been some kind of misdiagnosis or that the illness will turn out to be curable.
2 As time passes, patients move to the second phase where hope for successful treatment predominates.
3 People may move to a third phase of hope when they are told that nothing more can be done to cure them. Hope is then focused on prolongation of life.
4 Finally, hope for a peaceful death is the main concern. Hope becomes centred on the relief of physical symptoms, the maintenance of dignity and the wish to be loved and forgiven. Hope for some kind of afterlife may form part of this final phase.

Health professionals can begin the process of communication by listening and asking open questions that will help to elicit the patient's hope. Our role should be to alleviate their fears by giving appropriate information and support and by the assurance that we will meet any problems together. Dying people and their relatives need to know that we are as interested and skilled in their palliative care as we were when there was a possibility of cure.

Inappropriate information or too much information may

remove a person's hope by creating a gap between their expectations and reality. Truth that only emphasises the terminal nature of the illness takes away hope and leads to despair. Many writers have stressed the role of explanations and psychological support in alleviating patients' and relatives' anxieties about the effects of a terminal illness and its treatment. Such support is as essential as the medical treatment itself.

It is easy for doctors and nurses to forget that patients and relatives may be worrying unnecessarily about the effects of drugs such as diamorphine, or that they may fear the imagined consequences of the spread of the disease to other parts of the body. It is equally easy for doctors and nurses to overlook the extent to which patients can naturally give support to each other, since they are often best placed to empathise with someone in a similar position to their own.

Skilled support involves giving information when it is perceived to be needed by patients or relatives and being alert to situations when patients and relatives may be anxious. Too much information may provoke as much anxiety as too little, and it should always be tailored to the individual's needs.

Information should be given in a way that is not unduly negative or falsely reassuring. Buckman (1992) suggests a simple phrase: 'We'll plan for the worst but hope for the best'. This enables people to see that both are possible at the same time. Change is about looking for new options and giving up the old. Nurses can communicate this change of emphasis by their attitude to patients without making false promises. Nurses can encourage patients to set themselves short-term goals and plan with patients how to use their time and energy most effectively.

Quality of life

The experience of the hospice movement has shown that terminally ill people can have a fairly good quality of life in the time left to them if their own attitudes and those of the caring professionals remain positive. Relatives can be left with memories of hopes and love shared because communication has been open and honest. Dying people, often even more so than relatives, have great fears of losing dignity and of not coping and they need the reassurance of knowing that professional staff will not be afraid to listen to their fears and be available to them throughout the illness, even when they cannot solve all the problems. Providing comfort is essentially about acceptance and can be conveyed in practice by touch and by attending to every detail of physical care. Whenever possible, relatives can be involved in promoting comfort for the patient which may also bring them closer to each other. A relative of a hospice patient described his anxieties about his mother's terminal illness:

> 'From my point of view, home care was a load off my mind because I had visions of me struggling away with her lying dying in bed and me trying to cope with it. I imagined the hospice would be an austere place with people lying in bed and moaning and that sort of thing, and shouting out. It's not like that at all.'

The son quoted above went on to describe how his mother enjoyed her visits from home to the day hospice where patients can become involved in a variety of activities and, more importantly, receive support from other patients and staff:

> 'When she was at home, she would sit for ages talking about the day hospice. I would sit and listen to her for a good hour or two. She seemed to enjoy the day hospice. Nine times out of ten there was a lady at the door when she arrived to welcome her. Then there was a wee bunch of flowers when she came away sometimes. These things make a difference.'

Quality of life seems to comprise something more than physical comfort and symptom control. An important element seems to be living actively and positively, until this is genuinely no longer possible. For example, some patients have attended the day hospice one week and enjoyed their time there, but have deteriorated rapidly and died before they could return the following week. Dying people can be encouraged and enabled to do the things they want, whenever possible, to make plans on a day-to-day basis and to celebrate important times such as birthdays and wedding anniversaries. Staff can encourage such planning and the shortness of time that may be left need not be a deterrent. Small things which seem unimportant when someone is terminally ill can in fact be very important to the person concerned. For example, dentures which no longer fit may increase problems of poor appetite or mouth discomfort. Having a faulty hearing aid quickly repaired may make a great difference to a person's ability to enjoy conversation with his or her family. People can be encouraged to maintain their social contacts by having flexible visiting hours and facilities for visitors to have light snacks and a place to relax or stay overnight if they wish. It is sometimes forgotten that being ill at home can be a lonely experience for the patient and the carer. The patient can become increasingly dependent and housebound, with the relative unable to leave them alone, as the following example shows:

'When he was in the house, he was sitting in a chair and all he could see was the tops of the tenements opposite. He knew the times of the planes coming over Calton Hill. There was nobody passing. In the hospice, he can see people coming and going and the children playing outside. He can speak to people, whereas in the house there was no conversation at all and latterly the only thing he and my mother could talk about was their experience of hospital.'

Staff can maintain a positive approach to improving a person's quality of life by encouraging patients and their families to make plans. We need to consider whether to take the initiative in suggesting to patients and relatives what can be done in this area. We will, however, only be in a position to do so if we know the patients and their relatives well enough to be aware of their wishes. Individual care and attention is very highly valued by patients and relatives. Relatives like to feel that the patient is special to the staff as well as to themselves, as the following comments show:

'The staff here have got a lot more time for individual care and attention. The staff here take time to talk to people and know what's going on.'

'You're making all those patients still remain individuals.'

Patients also express satisfaction with this individualised care and attention and the perceived availability and experience of staff increase their sense of security.

'He didn't worry too much about coming here because he'd get more attention, he said. He's quite happy, as happy as you can be.'

'Mother likes it here because it's more relaxed. The staff have got more time for individual care and attention.'

Attention to what may appear to be minor detail is most important in improving a person's sense of well being. For example, arranging for a haircut can be a great morale booster. We need to be aware of priorities as determined by the patients – people they wish to see, things they want to do, an important date or event in the future they wish to celebrate. If we are aware of people's priorities, we can help them use their limited energies and the short time remaining to maximum effect and create some happy memories for relatives. Good communication with dying people and their relatives has to be set in the context of a total relationship between them and the professional carers. The skill of the professional is in being able to establish these relationships in a much shorter timescale than normal. The emphasis must be on the essentials and on being as natural as one would be in forming relationships on a personal rather than a strictly professional basis. Caring attitudes are conveyed in so many ways other than words.

Recognising the dying person

In chronic illness, it is sometimes difficult to know when the terminal phase has been reached. Elderly people may suffer the effects of arteriosclerosis or Alzheimer's disease for many years before they die. This can pose problems for professional carers and place severe strains on relatives. Who makes the decisions about therapy, or about the resources which should be used in an endeavour to keep a chronically ill person at home? For the elderly chronically ill, as for any age group, the main consideration is to maintain quality of life for the person and caring relatives. This requires very skilled judgement and ongoing assessment of the medical condition and social circumstances, especially when a person suffers from a number of chronic conditions and the prognosis is uncertain. It is often difficult to steer a middle course between a 'fight to the last' approach and the attitude 'Don't treat anything too energetically in the elderly'.

A myocardial infarction, chest infection or further extension of an existing cerebrovascular accident may increase an existing debility, hasten death or cause sudden death. Dramatic changes in condition will be noticed by everybody, but less marked changes may only be noticed by experienced staff. The difficulties in recognising that a person is dying pose problems for communication and support. The patient may be anxious, yet uncertain of what is happening. It cannot be assumed that an elderly person will more readily accept the prospect of death than someone younger. Relatives may need to be helped to face the probability that the patient will die. They do not always notice or want to believe this. Often the relatives of older patients are elderly themselves and time and care should be taken to explain to them the changes that take place or are likely to occur. Hospital wards are often busy and understaffed and community nurses have heavy caseloads. The needs and feelings of the nursing staff may be overlooked or not considered important, yet they may have invested a lot of themselves in a relationship with a chronically ill patient and family over many months or years.

Younger people with long-term debilitating conditions are another group in whom it may be difficult to recognise that a terminal stage in the illness has been reached. For example, children infected by meningitis may survive the initial illness, against all odds, only to be left severely mentally handicapped. Children with cystic fibrosis are now surviving into their teens and twenties. Parents' hopes for children's recovery may be dashed and raised many times as they survive each crisis. Eventually, parents can become emotionally exhausted. They will need skilled psychological support in the months and years that follow and not just in the acute stages of the child's illness, to enable them to face a future in which they know that sudden deterioration and death can occur at any time.

Sudden death

When a person dies suddenly, the shock to relatives and friends will be great. Research has shown that lack of preparation for bereavement can lead to difficulties and a poor outcome (Bowlby 1981, Lindemann 1944, Murphy 1988).

Wright (1996) noted that death by road traffic or other forms of accident can cause more anger than does natural sudden death and people will ask whether the dead person suffered.

Bereaved people may be so shocked at the time of death that the full emotional impact may not be felt until weeks or months later. A prolonged stage of numbness or denial will make support extremely difficult for both friends and professional carers. It is important that reactions to sudden death are not just accepted at face value. A person who expresses very little emotion at the time may be the one who needs the most help later in coming to terms with bereavement.

Bereaved relatives, who may be in a state of shock, should have someone to accompany them home and a relative should not be alone at home when news of a death is received. The police have a policy of sending two officers to deliver the news of a sudden death, so that one officer can remain with the bereaved person, if necessary, until another friend or relative comes to help. Worden (1991) claimed that intervention should begin at the scene of death with help being offered positively in words such as, 'I'm here to help you'. As a counsellor in a hospital accident and emergency department, Wright (1996) noticed that experiences at the time of sudden death could have a powerful impact on the grieving process. Giving news of death to relatives over the phone can be traumatic. In Wright's experience, if the hospital where the death took place is quickly accessible, it is better to tell people when they arrive at the hospital. If they have to travel a long distance, it is essential to be honest over the phone, giving clear, concise information. Suicide can cause great anguish among friends and relatives. It often results in bereavement being more devastating than in other forms of death (Henley 1983). The friends and relatives of the dead person often have an irrational sense of guilt and need counselling support.

Recent years have seen the formation of self-help groups to support relatives bereaved after cot death and road traffic accidents. This indicates the great need of the bereaved for continuing understanding and emotional support.

Improving communication

Communication in palliative care constitutes a delicate network of interaction between patients, relatives and staff. Problems arise if there are failures at any point in the network. Our support to patients and families must be sensitive to their changing needs. We need to know when to remain in the background and when to assume a more positive role. As nurses, we are key people in the support network, often receiving the confidences of patients and meeting relatives on a daily basis. We also have to be aware of the needs of our own colleagues for support in the sometimes stressful task of caring for the terminally ill, giving them opportunities to talk to us and to share their feelings with us. Not infrequently among hospice staff and in groups of nurses and other professionals visiting the hospice on courses, I have found someone painfully reminded of a past experience of bereavement or a seriously ill relative.

Working in a team with other professionals is more rewarding when mutual respect and a readiness to listen to other people's points of view exist. It is easy, however, to become defensive about professional boundaries, and keeping other team members (doctors, community nurses or clergy) informed is hard work but essential if the physical, psychosocial and spiritual care of patients and their relatives is not to suffer. Of course, good communication with professional colleagues can greatly increase job satisfaction for nurses.

Questions and exercises

1 What is being done in your area to provide seamless hospital and community support to patients with a

terminal illness? Is there any way in which hospital and community liaison could be improved in your clinical area?

2 What forms of support are available to patients with advanced disease in your area? Have any of the following forms of support been considered:

- self-help groups
- professionally led support groups
- complementary therapies
- telephone help lines.

Can you think of other forms of support that would help your patients?

3 When a patient dies suddenly, how do you give the news to the relatives? How do you support the relatives? Which aspects of your support are most effective? In what ways could you and your colleagues improve your support?

4 What realistic encouragements can you give dying patients and their relatives to maintain hope and prevent despair? Look at a recent care plan. Think of any ways in which you could have better encouraged the patients and relatives to set themselves short-term goals and use their time and energy more effectively.

2

The needs of staff caring for terminally ill people

It seems to me that although the care of dying people and their relatives can be stressful to the professionals concerned, it can also be very rewarding. Each person's experience of stress in palliative care is different, depending on previous experiences of death or bereavement and established ways of coping with the emotions aroused by stress of any kind. I believe it is important to have some insight into our feelings and to be able to acknowledge when we are upset, rather than giving the appearance to colleagues and patients that nothing ever troubles us. Being professional and retaining the ability to support others does not, in my experience, mean being invulnerable to feeling sad or, on occasions, angry.

Stress is not always destructive. At an optimum level it provides a stimulation, challenge and incentive to improve standards of care. Palliative care provides just such a challenge to our skills and makes great demands on personal and professional resources. A person who is ill at ease working

with the dying may need considerable help and understanding from colleagues to face up to fears which may be
subconscious. Hospice staff are not immune to stress arising
from their work. Wilson (1985) found that hospice nurses
were no more or less susceptible to stress than nurses
working in other specialties. Caring for patients' emotional
needs was considered by hospice nurses to be more stressful
than physical care, and patients with emotional needs
received significantly less contact from these nurses than
those whose needs were purely physical. There are, in my
experience, very few patients whose needs are purely
physical, but there are patients whose psychological needs
place considerable demands on staff for support. Wakefield
(2000) noted that for nurses who regularly care for dying
patients, grief can be like a powder keg in that nurses may
not be aware of the effects of grief and may be expected to
carry on as normal once a patient has died. In my own
research (Lugton 1994), emotional involvement with patients
with breast cancer could leave health visitors feeling vulnerable. One health visitor had formed a close supportive relationship with a patient with advanced cancer. She described
her feelings:

'It's quite involving. You tend to think about it as you
come away as well. The visits can take quite some time.
In fact Alice has gone through a grief type reaction. I see
a big need there. Mind you it can be very draining.'

As nurses, we need to be aware of the distancing strategies
we can use in communication to protect ourselves from pain,
for example, by giving excessive reassurance, and talking to
other nurses instead of to patients or relatives. We need to be
aware of our own attitudes to death and dying. Wakefield
(2000) suggested that nurses involved in palliative care have
a need for 'relentless self-care'. She advocated that staff be
encouraged to take part in 'closure conferences', meetings

where those staff who were most involved in caring for the dead person are given an opportunity to talk and discuss their feelings of loss with others. Nurses should also be encouraged to ask questions about the patient's illness in order to 'make sense of events' and 'avoid self-blame for the person's death or the feeling that they had not done enough'. It is important to recognise that professional helpers, as well as patients and relatives, have needs in palliative care. Some of these needs are as follows:

1 being adequately prepared for work in palliative care and having the opportunities to gain skills and confidence
2 having the time, space and privacy to communicate with dying patients and their relatives
3 developing self-awareness and knowledge of their own attitudes and feelings
4 developing the qualities necessary for effective relationships with dying patients and their relatives
5 developing realistic expectations of what can be achieved
6 developing teamwork and receiving support from colleagues.

These needs will now be considered in more detail.

Being prepared for work in palliative care

Inadequate preparation for work in palliative care often results in a lack of confidence on the part of staff. According to Webber (1993), palliative care nursing demands three levels of competence. Level one of the model identifies competences, which can be expected of any registered nurse. Level two competences would be expected of nurses who have had a formal education or in-depth experience in palliative care. Level three competences are advanced. Describing Webber's model as it relates to communications, Kindlen and

Walker (1999) note that the competences expected of every registered nurse in order to assess and plan care are as follows:

- establish empathy
- listen
- give information
- assess needs, symptoms, psychosocial distress and the impact of these on the patient and family
- recognise situations where referral is required
- represent the patient's and family's needs to others.

Nurses working in the specialty of palliative care should be able to assess patients and families with identified psychological problems and assist them to explore distressing feelings utilising interventions to prevent psychological problems from developing or escalating. Advanced practitioners should be able to assess those with complex psychosocial problems and provide psychological support using a recognised therapeutic framework.

Attitudes influence every aspect of care – psychosocial, spiritual or physical. In the past, physical aspects of palliative care were overstressed in nursing education at the expense of the more difficult task of exploring emotions and attitudes. Thankfully, education in palliative care is improving, but many nurses and other professionals are still underprepared for all aspects of the work. Coping with death and dying is personally demanding and enabling nurses to overcome defensive attitudes is still a challenge. Mills *et al.* (1994) found that dying patients were left alone for long periods and received less attention from nurses than did other patients. Nurses' attitudes towards pain control and the use of opiates in palliative care will affect their skills and confidence in monitoring pain and in ensuring that adequate analgesia is given. If the use of opiates is equated with euthanasia, hastening of the patient's death or excessive drowsiness, there will be a reluctance to cooperate fully in using such drugs or in recognising the patient's need for them.

Palliative care can often be seen as unrewarding to health-care professionals because these patients do not get better. Too many doctors and nurses still regard a patient's death as a failure on their part. However, palliative care is increasingly recognised by professionals and by the general public as an area requiring special skills in symptom control and psycho-logical support and there has been a growth of specialist services in the community, hospitals and hospices. Courses in palliative care for the various healthcare professionals are now well established, at diploma, degree and masters levels. There are full-time courses, part-time courses and distance learning programmes. Research in palliative care has indi-cated ways to raise standards, and journal articles and books on the subject are now readily available. It is possible to develop our skills in communication and support as well as in the physical care of the dying. Counselling courses, both specialised and general, of varying lengths and intensity are widely available; for example, CRUSE, a national organisation for the bereaved (*see* Appendix: Useful addresses) runs courses for its volunteer counsellors.

Creating time, space and privacy for communication

It is important to create an atmosphere of space and privacy to talk with and listen to dying people and their relatives. At the hospice, nurses with a general hospital background often complained that there was nowhere private to go in a busy ward. Often there were frequent interruptions and telephone calls, which occurred just at the moment when a patient or relative was trying to express his or her deepest anxieties and fears. This makes it very difficult to have anything but very hurried and superficial conversations with patients and relatives.

A room apart, which provides privacy and freedom from interruptions, can be a great asset and should not be impossible to obtain if there is real concern about giving patients and relatives the opportunities to talk which they have the right to expect. Nurses often feel guilty about spending time in this way because the results of such communications are not always apparent and some of the information may be given in confidence. Two comfortable chairs placed close to each other at a ninety-degree angle should enable a patient or relative to feel relaxed. The environment in which we conduct such a discussion should convey the respect we wish to show to the patient or relative. Some hospitals now have rooms which are furnished so that relatives can stay overnight or at least doze in an armchair when visiting a very sick person. This helps to convey a feeling that the needs of the relative are considered to be important to hospital staff. When talking to patients who are in bed, it is better for staff to sit in a chair by the bed so that they are not looking down on the patient or appearing to be in a hurry to get away. At home, there is generally more privacy for patients than in hospital but sometimes a person has too many well-meaning friends and neighbours calling and feels exhausted as a result. The community nurse may have to make tactful suggestions about the best visiting arrangements for the patient.

Self-awareness in palliative care

Personal experiences can influence attitudes to work with dying people, e.g. witnessing a painful death, or having a difficult bereavement. Sometimes carers are not aware of how much such an experience still affects them until situations at work remind them of their own loss. The experience of losing a close relative or friend can give staff added insight and sensitivity in working with dying and bereaved people, but it is easy to underestimate personal needs in our anxiety to help others. We need to understand our own emotions and to acknowledge them and to act on the advice that we often give to the bereaved, not to suppress feelings or pretend that we are always coping. Self-awareness from reflective practice is at the core of developing communication and counselling skills in palliative care. Self-awareness is one of the qualities that Carkuff (1969) considered necessary in effective counselling. Other qualities were empathy, genuineness and unconditional acceptance of others. A climate of trust is created not only by what is said but also by the understanding shown in facial expression, tone of voice and gestures. These demonstrate our confidence in the person and their ability to use their own resources to help themselves. Egan (1990) noted that skilled helpers are able to explore their own behaviour and know what it means to be helped. This self-knowledge can help them avoid or cope with burn out. They are aware of the emotions with which they are comfortable and those in themselves or others which give them trouble.

Dying people and their relatives evoke the normal range of feelings in the staff who are caring for them. Staff may feel unable to express any negative feelings about people because they are dying. This may not be helpful either to patients or their relatives. Bereaved people often feel they can no longer acknowledge the faults and failings of the deceased and this in turn can give rise to feelings of guilt over their own attitudes and behaviour. Relationships within a family can become distorted if relatives feel that the dying person can never be contradicted. The patient may feel unsafe with staff who are 'too kind' since he or she may feel unable to express their own negative emotions. Nurses should behave as human beings with human emotions and should not only be concerned with appearing clinically correct.

It is important to monitor the development of our skills in

supporting the terminally ill and their relatives. Sometimes we are conscious of using these skills, for example, when we have successfully interpreted non-verbal cues as to how a patient is feeling. At other times we are equally conscious of having failed to understand or communicate with them sensitively. It can be very revealing when we assess our interactions with patients and relatives on a day-to-day basis. Discovering our own needs and motivations is an ongoing process, requiring courage and honesty. In this way we build up a picture of our own strengths and weaknesses as communicators. Personal growth can be maintained by a willingness to learn from real life situations (a kind of 'critical incident' technique). There are also support and growth groups which provide opportunities to benefit from the insights of others.

Developing necessary qualities

For effective relationships with patients and their relatives, a professional and personal approach is required. The personal relationships developed in palliative care, which are essential to giving patients and relatives adequate support, may mean that from time to time we get over-involved or identify too closely with a particular patient or relative. Staff can identify strongly with certain patients, e.g. patients of their own age, those who remind them of someone close to them, or those with attractive personalities. There is a need to develop such personal relationships with patients in palliative care to understand and support them. The relationship often has within it elements of friendship. The key to effective support is availability and being ready at any time and in any way to respond to the needs of the patient. Many people imagine that care of dying people is always depressing and stressful. A theology student on a course at the hospice describes how his views were changed:

'One of my main feelings before working at the hospice was an uneasiness with the presence of death. I did not feel able to cope with the bereaved person, having no idea how to help them. My hospice experience radically altered that. I came to realise that by my contact with the patients, dying was not the catastrophic ending I thought it might be. I learned that care required a large range of responses, the ability to listen, the ability not to interfere, coupled with complete willingness to be available and to be turned away.'

Dying patients, like other people, want us to respond to them in a natural way. They do not want us always to be solemn and are almost always able to share a smile or appreciate a joyful event. Getting close to patients is one of the most rewarding aspects of palliative care, but we cannot mourn the death of each patient as we would that of a close relative or friend. Care should be taken in nursing practice that empathy is not confused with identification. Empathy enables the helper to put themselves in another's position and to recognise how that person may be feeling. Identification means that the helper becomes the other person to the extent of taking on his or her problems. The patient or relative needs to be helped to work through their own anxieties and problems. Therefore, helpers must remain themselves to be effective for patients and relatives and to ensure their own survival.

Developing realistic expectations

Staff may have unrealistic expectations of what can be accomplished in palliative care. This is the opposite of the attitude 'there's nothing more that can be done'. For example, nurses are often idealistic, committed to their work, and find they are sometimes unable to meet the standards they have set themselves. They may be unable to spend as much time as they would like with patients when short staffed. Nurses from large NHS hospitals or with heavy caseloads in the community, often see the principles of care espoused by the hospice movement as unattainable in their own situation. It is important that nurses' expectations of themselves are realistic, otherwise they may defend themselves from anxiety by remaining emotionally detached from patients and relatives and concentrating on physical care.

In spite of every effort by doctors or nurses, some patients are depressed or have a very poor quality of life. Staff may be disturbed by their apparent inability to control symptoms or give dying patients the emotional support they are seeking. Some patients have a fear of death rather than the experience of dying and can be very difficult to help, as hospice Examples 2.1 and 2.2 show.

Example 2.1

'She's worried about herself, the thought of dying. She doesn't say much. She keeps a lot to herself. When she sees the rest of them, she sees a lot of pitiful sights. Every time they close her door she knows there's another body going past. She knows that because when she was in hospital one of the nurses said, "I'll have to close the door. It's an old man that's died". She's frightened. She told the doctor she just wished it were all over.'

Example 2.2

'It was a very traumatic business for her to decide to come in. She knows all too well that this is it in terms of her illness. She's not happy, but who is happy in the terminal stages of lung cancer. I don't think it's anything to do with the hospice, her unhappiness. All the staff are very kind.'

Some people, in the past, have had distressing experiences which make it difficult for them to accept support when it is offered in the last few weeks of life. The concept of 'good enough care', as described by Winnicot (1965) in regard to mothering can be helpful in setting realistic expectations for patient care. No mother can hope to meet every need of her baby. In a similar way we cannot meet every need of dying patients or overcome all the constraints imposed by our work situations. Acceptance of our limitations will enable us to discard guilt over not being able to solve other peoples' problems. All that we can offer is help to enable patients and relatives to cope better themselves.

Developing teamwork and receiving support

Nurses can be very unsupported in their care of dying and bereaved people. This lack of support can occur at all levels of the profession, from student nurses to senior staff. In theory, a multiprofessional team harnesses skills required for the task in a unique way which would be impossible outside the team (Øvretveit 1995). The multiprofessional team has a number of advantages:

- an increased range of services
- the workload is easier to manage
- collegiate support
- cross fertilisation of ideas
- a more holistic approach.

The team's ability to make decisions is affected by the way in which the members communicate. The involvement of all members is vital to solving complex problems and will result in high-quality decisions being made. Honesty and mutual respect are important in team building. However, Plant's (1987) 'iceberg model' of the team notes that organisations often resemble icebergs in having hidden, invisible, areas under the surface which can influence organisational development. Traditionally, hospitals have had a hierarchical culture with a top down medical-led approach to organising work. This can militate against successful team working. In contrast hospices have valued a multiprofessional approach stressing equality. Hospital palliative care teams have had difficulty in introducing hospice philosophy into an acute, cure-focused, organisation (Hockley and Dunlop 1990). Role identification was easy for medical staff and social workers but nurses found this more difficult. This may be because the role of the clinical nurse specialist overlaps most with medical and social work roles (Hockley and Dunlop 1990). In palliative care, the concept of desirable role blurring, as identified by Ajeman (1995), has yet to be resolved within hospital palliative care teams. Sofaer (1983) showed the importance of mutual communication between doctors and nurses in achieving pain control in surgical wards. Nurses too readily accept that the prime responsibility for achieving good symptom control is medical. However, confrontational methods of communication between nurses and doctors are not helpful in resolving problems for the patient's benefit. For example, nurses should accept responsibility in reporting a patient's pain and in monitoring the effects of analgesics. The patient's assessment of pain control using a pain chart may be more objective, detailed and less opinionated than the nurse's 'view' on the patient's drug regime.

The importance of good communication and cooperation among healthcare professionals was recognised in the Calman and Hine report (1995) which emphasised early integration of palliative care services. Community nurses will recognise the importance of good communication between themselves and the hospital when a patient is discharged home. Unfortunately, the accompanying note often details the diagnosis and treatment given but gives no indication of what the patient and relatives have been told about the illness or prognosis. Until the note from the hospital arrives explaining the position or a telephone call is made to the ward, the primary care team may be in the embarrassing position of trying to discover what the patient and family know. In this interval, damage can be done, as the nurse will know the diagnosis and, possibly by non-verbal communication, gives the patient cause for concern.

The support of colleagues in the professional team is essential. Colleagues can provide valuable opportunities for nurses to talk about their own feelings and experiences with the terminally ill. However, opportunities need to be created if such support is to be available, so team meetings and case conferences are important in this regard. Support groups may be useful for staff working in more isolated situations. Junior staff should be given structured opportunities to talk to their seniors about their experiences with dying patients and their relatives. It is important that such opportunities are created in the clinical situation as well as in the academic institution. Staff may have had distressing personal experiences of death and bereavement which will affect their attitudes to palliative care unless they are given opportunities to share their anxieties and receive support. Senior staff can sometimes act as role models for students, for example, in taking a student with them when talking to a patient or relative whenever possible. The psychological privacy of patients and relatives should always be respected and it is not necessary to reveal to the whole team confidences given to a particular staff member who has developed a close relationship with a patient and family.

Cultivating mutual respect between professionals is essential if colleagues are to support each other and give support to dying people and their relatives. This may be achieved for example, through regular team meetings, case conferences and interdisciplinary education which enable the various professionals to see more clearly the contribution each can make and to become more aware of the dilemmas each may encounter at work. Staff are supported when members of the different caring professions share knowledge of what can be achieved in palliative care and are in agreement about the ways in which patients can be helped.

Recognition and support come not only from colleagues but perhaps surprisingly, from dying people, patients and their relatives. They are, after all, part of the team. They can teach us so much about the experience of dying and bereavement and often cope with their difficulties with great courage. They encourage us to reflect on the meaning of life and often help us to put our smaller personal problems into perspective. Dying patients are often flatteringly grateful for anything that is done for their well being. This should not prevent us from always seeking to improve our care.

Some ways in which we can reduce the stress involved in palliative care have been described in this chapter. I believe that we should be prepared to make periodic self-assessments and review our work with colleagues so that we can maintain a fresh and sensitive approach and develop new skills in this important area. Sometimes frustrations and stresses in palliative care seem to be beyond our control as, for example, in the experience of professional isolation or lack of support from colleagues. It is important to identify the constraints within a situation, but also to be aware of opportunities and possibilities for change. Nurses working in busy hospitals or in the community have often seen hospices as 'ideal' situations and have pointed out the difficulties of applying the principles of hospice care in their own work settings where they are less well staffed, or where they work with colleagues who do not seem to share their views about palliative care. Many of these nurses have found it productive to consider one or two aspects of palliative care over which they have influence and wish to improve, rather than seeking to make too many changes in the short term. For example, a Macmillan nurse decided to concentrate on improving communications between her colleagues and the district nurses in her area. There is, in my opinion, almost always something that we can do to improve the care of dying patients and their relatives.

Questions and exercises

1 Nurses involved in palliative care have a need for 'relentless self-care'. What strategies do/could you use as an individual to take care of yourself? What self-care strategies does/could your professional team use?
2 Support for terminally ill people demands three levels of competence (Webber 1993). How confident do you feel in your own level of competence? What do you do best? How could you improve your support skills?
3 What emotions in yourself or others are comfortable? What emotions in yourself and others give you trouble? How could you improve the way you cope with difficult emotions in yourself or in a patient or relative?
4 In what ways have you tried to monitor your communication skills? Would you consider any of the following methods of evaluation helpful?
   • Tape-recorded/video-recorded interview (e.g. with a colleague).
   • Discussion of your support of individual patients at a team meeting or case conference.
   • Retrospective self-evaluation of your interactions with particular patients and relatives.

3

Breaking bad news

In communicating the diagnosis of a terminal illness or a poor prognosis, most medical and nursing staff are likely to have experienced problems. Feelings of inadequacy, concern about the patient's reactions, together with the constraints of team policy on giving information, may result in nurses avoiding rather than facing up to the issues.

Assessing patients' awareness and reactions

It is important to explore patients' awareness of and reactions to their own terminal illness in order to assess their need for further information or support. Research has shown that patients often know they have a serious illness, even when they have not been explicitly told. Nursing experience confirms this. We may well be aware that a patient is anxious because they suspect they have cancer.

In the past there was a practice by the professionals of non-disclosure of bad news to the patient although relatives were often informed. A study by McIntosh (1977) showed how patients responded differently to information about their illness. Some people wanted more information while others were content with the minimum level to enable them to cope with their situation. In McIntosh's study, 88% of patients knew or suspected that they had cancer but most did not want further information. McIntosh felt that those who wanted to know more would ask. Seale (1991) commented that forcing the truth on those who do not want or cannot cope with it could be just as inexcusable as avoiding honest discussion. Commenting on his study of the terminal care of older dying patients in hospital, Costello (2000) maintained that nurses working in palliative care settings should answer patients' questions as honestly as possible whilst remembering that telling the patient the whole truth may sometimes be insensitive and uncaring.

There appear to be cultural differences in approaches to truth telling. The Ad Hoc Committee on Medical Ethics (1984) in the USA indicated that it is a duty for physicians to tell patients when they are dying. However, in Japan there has been a tradition of telling the relatives the diagnosis while protecting the patient from the bad news. In a Japanese study (Seo *et al.* 2000) the aim was to clarify patients', physicians' and nurses' perceptions with regard to the communication of diagnosis to cancer patients. Of 63 patients, 54 wished to be informed of the diagnosis. Physicians did not tell the truth to the remaining patients of whom seven were not told the diagnosis because family members objected. Of the 35 physicians, 21 thought that telling the true diagnosis had a positive effect and 27 thought that disclosure of the diagnosis to cancer patients should be promoted. Sixteen of the 21 nurses did not experience any difficulties with patient care after the diagnosis was disclosed. The study suggested that medical staff and family members should respect the patient's standpoint because patients have the right to know about their condition. In the UK there have now been moves towards full disclosure. People are also more questioning about their illnesses and treatment and many people use the Internet to get the information they seek. However, Katz and Sidell (1994) noted that although many patients want information about a terminal diagnosis, some institutions or departments still refrain from full disclosure. Penson (1990) reported that, even when information about dying is disclosed, it is usually given in more optimistic terms to the patient than to the relatives.

Many patients are reticent about asking medical staff or 'busy' nurses for information, unless they are given explicit opportunities to talk about their suspicions and fears. If patients are anxious and are not given explanations of their condition or treatment, they may imagine something far more frightening than the reality. They and their families may need considerable help along the road to knowledge and ultimately towards a peaceful death.

Assessing coping styles and planning support

It is important to explore patients' awareness of, and reactions to, their own terminal illness in order to assess their need for further information or support. Unfortunately, people often become defensive and their behaviour less adaptable when under threat. When a person is diagnosed with a terminal illness, his or her reactions to the diagnosis can be extreme (Buckman 1995).

Defensiveness in the face of actual or suspected bad news is a necessary, and even helpful, response in patients and relatives because it helps them to maintain a degree of hopefulness for the future and gives patients the opportunity to take the lead in asking for information. As discussed earlier, total truth, presented in an uncompromising manner, can be as damaging to patients and relatives as a conspiracy of silence by professionals.

We need to be able to identify each patient's coping style

and its possible consequences. For example, denial of the seriousness of the situation may be helpful to patients in the earlier stages of their illness because it helps them to cope with surgery or unpleasant chemotherapy. If denial continues, however, it may mean that communication within the family becomes blocked and members are left unsupported in their anxiety. Kubler Ross (1970) described five reactions to impending loss, i.e. denial, anger, bargaining, depression and acceptance. I would add anxiety as being an emotion experienced by most patients at different stages of their terminal illness. Relatives can react to impending bereavement in a similar way, although, as the patient's experience draws to a close, the relatives' experience is just beginning. Lewis (1961) described his feelings when his wife was dying of cancer:

> *'I had my miseries, not hers; she had hers, not mine. The end of hers would be the coming of age of mine. We were setting out on different roads. This cold truth, this terrible traffic regulation ("you, madam to the right – you, sir, to the left") is just the beginning of the separation, which is death itself.'*

Stages in coping with advanced disease

The stages in coping with terminal illness, as described by Kubler Ross, can be interpreted too literally. Some patients, for example, may appear to pass through a stage of denial to one of acceptance, but when further signs of the advance of the disease appear, they may deny the deterioration. There is also a danger in regarding all defences as essentially bad when in fact they may be helping particular individuals to cope in a time of great personal stress. It can be particularly difficult in a long illness to maintain the fine balance between hope and reality, so that the patient does not fall into despair.

For example, it may be envisaged that a patient with motor neurone disease will soon require a wheelchair, which has been adjusted to their needs. The order for the wheelchair has to be placed considerably in advance of when it is actually needed. The difficulty for staff is getting the patient to accept that the wheelchair will ultimately be required when their condition deteriorates, while at the same time maintaining their present confidence and independence. So patients reach a point in their illness when they are neither depressed nor angry at their fate. This stage of acceptance is not the same as giving up in the sense of being unable to fight any longer. Kubler Ross (1970) describes the stage of acceptance as follows:

'Acceptance should not be mistaken for a happy stage. It is almost void of feelings. It is as if the pain had gone, the struggle is over and there comes a time for "the final rest before the long journey" as one patient phrased it. It is also a time during which the family usually needs more help, understanding and support than the patient himself.'

Some of the reactions to impending loss and the implications for support of patients and relatives are now considered.

Denial – acceptance

Denial can offer protection from the threat of disintegration that might come with complete loss of hope. It can represent a rational and vital buffer against hopelessness. A person who is using denial as a means of coping, discourages others from giving him information about his illness because he wishes to make his situation appear less frightening to himself. Careful, sensitive, listening by professionals is essential (Lugton 1994). One of my patients, Angela, coped with having advanced cancer by putting her illness to the back of her mind. She was not helped in this by her GP.

> *'It's like being in limbo. It's been like that for two years. When you think you've got over one bit, something else crops up (crying). For a long time I worried, then it sort of dawned on me that I was still here. You could put it in the background. Then that stupid doctor made me feel it was going to be my last Christmas. I wouldn't even see January. From then on it was difficult.'*

When a person's condition deteriorates it becomes more difficult to deny the reality of the situation. Patients and relatives need to talk to nurses openly about their fears and if we allow them to persist too long in denial, problems may not be aired and anxieties will increase. It is important to make an accurate assessment of any sources of anxiety. However, truth should be given gently and there is a need to maintain hope. If we are confident and hopeful in our approach to palliative care this will elicit hope in the patient. Herth (1990) maintained that hope can operate as a significant coping force within a close relationship and evidence of hope in one person has a role in sustaining hopefulness in another. Herth's hope-fostering strategies were meaningful shared relationships, lightheartedness, courage, attainable aims, spiritual beliefs and affirmation of worth.

Sometimes relatives have not fully accepted the person's terminal illness although they are aware of the diagnosis. In the hospice, one man was holding on to the hope that his wife had been admitted for observation and would be going home:

> *'This is the place that's got the name for careful monitoring of any patient, so I was very relieved to get her in here. Are there any other patients in here for*

monitoring? I know that most of them are seriously ill. I thought that was all you dealt with here.'

One woman had accepted that her husband had a terminal illness, but not the very short prognosis:

'It's terrible to sort of really know but not want to know. Dave's voice started to go since last Monday and I didn't know it was the illness that was causing it. I thought, "He's been talking too much". I didn't twig. I didn't realise that the pain in the back is pressure from this tumour. I thought Dave would be in here a year or two years.'

Anger

Seriously ill people and their relatives may show a lot of anger or aggression. Often this disguises underlying fears and anxieties. If a patient's anger is directed against relatives and friends or caring professionals, it may discourage them from trying to help, thus leaving the person lonely and isolated. Sometimes anger shows itself in constant complaints about treatment and care. Looked at from the patient's or relatives' perspective there sometimes seems to be good reason for the anger – perhaps there was a delay in making a diagnosis, or treatment was extremely unpleasant and did not cure the patient. Unresolved anger may prevent the dying person and their family from using the time that remains to them positively.

Patients' and relatives' anger can be defused to some extent if they are able to talk freely about their experiences and difficulties, and when they feel satisfied that staff are accepting and trying to understand their feelings. Examples 3.1 and 3.2 illustrate these two points.

Example 3.1

'On Tuesday (prior to her mother's hospice admission), I phoned someone here. I don't know who it was. I spoke to her and I think I poured out my heart to her. I was just so cross with the GP. I felt better after it. Mum has really been ill for a long time. They forgot about her in hospital and it's really an awful story. The file was just lying in a basket. The GP didn't visit unless we called him.'

Example 3.2

'I suppose they were a bit rushed in the hospital but she was in great pain and she wanted something. She was given the impression "Why do you need to disturb us?"'

It can be very difficult for staff to cope with anger when it is directed at them, even when they sense that it is an outer manifestation of a patient's fears and uncertainties. Being too defensive is probably not very helpful. We may have to acknowledge actual shortcomings in our care, if, for example, they occurred through shortage of staff, and convey to the patient that we are trying to understand their difficulties. Anger may cause problems to patients in their illness and to relatives during bereavement, if it leads them to brood over what might have been. Relatives' anger may be expressed at professionals or even at the deceased for leaving them to cope with life alone. Aspects of the reality that is creating the anger should be explored and expectations about care and treatment discussed to see to what extent they are realistic and can be met or what alternatives are open. Physical activity can be an effective, non-verbal means of expressing pent-up emotion. An outing, or involvement in craftwork, can provide such an outlet.

Bargaining

When they realise that their illness is terminal, some patients and their relatives try to bargain with medical staff or with God for a cure or a remission. Staff may find it difficult to respond positively since they do not wish either to encourage unrealistic expectations or to destroy patients' and relatives' hopes. This is a time when patients may seek advice about alternative therapies or about alterations to their diet or healing through prayer. We should not discourage patients from exploring these areas, but help them to reach their own decisions about what is right for them, unless we are aware that they are embarking on a harmful course of action. Not taking decision making away from terminally ill patients is particularly important because they may be struggling to maintain some sort of control over their lives and are often all too conscious that their independence is slipping away.

Depression

While the assumption that all dying people are depressed is not true, a significant proportion do suffer from depression. Depression is associated with actual or anticipated losses. Serious illness involves many kinds of loss (Lugton 1994). There is loss of independence, physical attractiveness, role relationships and ultimately life itself. The significance of each loss depends, of course, on the individual concerned, but can be mitigated by the support received. Important indicators of depression are feelings of hopelessness, loss of self-esteem, guilt and wishing to die (Billings 1995). An association has been found between multiple distressing symptoms and depression and this accords with my clinical experience. For example, mood disturbance is closely related to increased pain (Zimmerman *et al.* 1996). Spiritual and emotional difficulties are often closely linked. For example, a patient whose feelings of guilt are making him depressed may be helped by a talk with the chaplain or clergyman.

Only a small proportion of depression among terminally ill people is diagnosed and treated appropriately (Brietbart *et al.* 1995). The lack of appropriate treatment can intensify other symptoms and affect the patient's quality of life. Much current research suggests that psychiatric consultation is a valuable asset in the management of depression in terminally ill patients. In reality, this consultation does not occur very often (Finnannon 1995). We should not accept depression as an inevitable part of dying, but explore its causes so that we can give appropriate support. Management of depression is focused upon reducing emotional distress, improving morale, regaining a sense of control and the resolution of problems (Massie *et al.* 1994). It is important to review patients' psychological state at regular intervals, approaching patients directly about how they are feeling and waiting for the reply. Maguire (1995) suggested that health professionals tend to offer premature reassurance, thus denying patients the opportunity to express all their concerns and preventing the detection of psychological problems. Many experienced nurses will know that peaceful and even happy deaths do occur and can leave a lasting impression on relatives, friends and staff. Social interaction is important in depression therapy. If family and carers are unable to provide such support the patient is unlikely to achieve peace of mind. Twycross (1995) suggested that encouraging patients to attend day centres helps to provide the social integration required as part of their therapy.

Anxiety

Most terminally ill patients and their relatives are anxious about the future and some show extreme anxiety. Patients may be anxious about frightening symptoms such as pain or dyspnoea, about becoming confused or losing control and dignity (*see* Chapter 4). Some patients are afraid of death and may be unable to sleep because of fears of dying at this time. Distressing symptoms can make a person feel unsafe at home and can be a reason for admission to a hospice or hospital, as the following example shows:

'Soon after she was in, I saw she was more relaxed. She says "I've still got the pain, but it's not so dreadful, and I'm not afraid because I know people will help me".'

Patients may feel unable to cope with treatment such as chemotherapy because of its distressing side effects, yet be afraid that their illness will progress rapidly if treatment is stopped, as the following example illustrates:

'What frightened Margaret was the thought that it was the end and the hospice wouldn't do anything for her. Her own doctor said "We could take you into the hospice", but she said "No", so they took her into the hospital and she got more treatment there.'

Relatives are naturally anxious about the patient's daily condition but also worry about how they will cope with the terminal illness and with their own bereavement (*see* Chapter 6). The responsibility of caring for dying people at home and ensuring, for example, that they do not fall, can be exhausting for relatives. The cumulative effect of being almost continuously with a sick person takes its toll, as the following examples show.
    A daughter describes caring for her mother at home:

'You're sort of worried about her all the time. Everything just seemed to get on top of me. My sisters have been upset and I've been upset, but I've been the one that's had to carry them along.'

A son was anxious about the effects of his father's illness on his mother:

'She'd rarely leave the house. Really she had 23 hours a day with him and some very bad nights when he was restless. Nothing too dramatic but a lot to live with all the time.'

When a dying person is living alone, this is usually a concern to relatives even if they are living nearby, and is often a contributory factor in hospital or hospice admission.

'My sister and I were worried especially at night. I wanted to be there in case she was in pain. She was on her own at night and that was the biggest worry.'

The most helpful factor in alleviating anxiety in patients and relatives is a professional who is well known and trusted and whose judgement is respected, hence the need for early involvement of the district nurse and/or Macmillan nurse. Patients can feel secure in hospital or a hospice, even if their distressing symptoms are not completely controlled, if they feel confident in the staff. Very anxious relatives may be helped to cope by involvement in the patient's nursing care. Nurses should take the initiative in suggesting this, when they consider that it may be helpful. Patients and relatives should be encouraged to talk about any nebulous fears they have in a more specific way. Often it is not so much the thought of death that makes patients afraid as fear of dying, or anxiety about some imagined effect of their disease, such as choking or suffocating or having uncontrolled pain. When the patient or relatives have expressed more precisely the nature of their anxieties, it is often possible for the nurse to give genuine reassurance.

Obsessional behaviour

Some dying patients develop a tendency to obsessional behaviour, such as noting down all the details of their treatment or tidying the contents of a bedside locker. Obsessional behaviour may be an effort on the patient's part to regain control of the situation.

Supporting the patient's identity in advanced illness

In a crisis such as advanced illness, a redefinition of the self-concept may become necessary and much encouragement from professionals and family may be needed to make this shift possible. It is often difficult for people to maintain adequate concepts of self when undergoing changes caused by serious illness (Anderson 1988a,b, Kelly 1991, Lugton 1994, Tait 1988). The degree to which an illness affects the individual's core identities varies from person to person but people who are ill are likely to face several identity crises.

Support is a concept, which is frequently but vaguely used in nursing. My own research into the experiences of women with breast cancer indicated that the underlying essence of support is the way in which it maintains individuals' identities and their sense of self (Lugton 1994). In some circumstances, support also helps people to adapt their self-perceptions to their changed circumstances.

Support from family, friends and fellow patients

Informal support from family, friends and fellow patients helps women with breast cancer to cope with anxiety, fear and depression in seven important ways (Lugton 1997):

- emotional support
- companionship
- practical help
- opportunities for confiding
- peer support (from other patients)
- support for sexual identity (especially by partners)
- advocacy (e.g. accompanying patients to clinic appointments).

As nurses we should aim to help people maintain and, if necessary, create their own informal support during illness. This is explored more fully in Chapter 5.

Professional support

Professional support is important. The process of protecting and building patients' identities starts with careful assessment of the person. Important questions are:

- How is this person feeling?
- What important aspects of this person's identity (including significant relationships, future plans, important roles) are threatened by the present situation?

Serious illness and people's core identities

Some of the ways in which serious illness can affect people's core identities are now considered and associated professional support discussed.

Uncertainty/insecurity

Being in control of one's life is an important aspect of identity. For this, predictability is necessary. In my research in a breast cancer unit, women faced an uncertain future (Lugton 1994). Anxiety about recurrence made them suspicious of any aches and pains they experienced. Because of cancer's association in society with death, they were stopped in their tracks. It was a threat to the very core of their self. Health visitors helped patients to cope with their fears, not with false reassurance, but by encouraging them to talk about their anxieties and by providing appropriate medical information. Anne, who had advanced cancer, was unwilling to confide in her family but appreciated her health visitor's approach:

'She's very important. She's at the hub (of contacts). She's easy to talk to. She doesn't feel like a health visitor. She's the person I talk to most. She's sympathetic but not too sympathetic because I can't take that.'

Another patient, Linda, also valued the opportunity to speak to a professional person outside her family circle:

'It's nice to speak to someone totally outside the family. I suppose people you know quite well can be frightened to say the wrong things or know how to react. I think some are a bit wary about what to say and what not to say.'

Putting the illness into perspective

It is important for their quality of life that people with advanced disease are able to put their illness into perspective so that it does not completely dominate their lives. Joan, who had a recurrence of her breast cancer, spoke of being unexpectedly vulnerable in the period after her mastectomy four years previously:

'Up to then I'd never really been ill. I felt it had done quite a bit to me, physically and I was not quite the same person. After I'd had the mastectomy, I really did feel ill, if not ill, at least physically less able to do things than I had been. I felt very vulnerable at first going out and doing things.'

We can help patients to do this by encouraging them to explore their feelings openly and to think positively about palliative treatments, which may be able to alleviate their symptoms. Such treatment can enable people with advanced disease to remain in control of their lives. Joan was grateful for a reasonable quality of life:

'It was diagnosed there in the tummy, a secondary. I had these pills for a while. I had these jags for about eighteen months. It seems to have kept it at bay, which is great. I'm grateful to be here all these years.'

There are problems of maintaining hope despite a poor prognosis and availability of support is important in this. Health visitors with extra training in breast cancer care were perceived to be very helpful by patients (Lugton 1994). Rose's health visitor was a medically knowledgeable 'outsider' with whom she could discuss her anxieties:

'She came the day after I was told (recurrence). It's someone other than a friend, somebody with a bit of knowledge who doesn't laugh at you. I know that if I did need help in any way, she has got connections.'

Dependence

In advanced illness, physical limitations may mean that physical dependence increases as the disease progresses.

Lynam's (1990) research into the support of young adults with lymphoma and sarcoma emphasised the importance to their identity of their ability to fulfil social roles. All her respondents defined who they were in terms of their social roles and relationships and the feelings derived from them. In my research many women treated for breast cancer worried about their competence to carry out normal social and work roles (Lugton 1994). Many found themselves temporarily, and a few permanently, unable to cope. Inability to carry out normal social and work roles can affect self-esteem. One woman who had had bilateral mastectomies was surprised at how tired and old she felt.

> 'The tiredness surprises me. I was one of those lucky people, you know. I had loads of energy. I could cope with my job, my housework and everything without feeling tired. Now by the time I've washed and dressed in the morning and sat down, I can feel my eyes getting heavy. You think, "Gosh I feel like somebody of ninety".'

Celia, who had advanced breast cancer, had to take time off for hospital appointments. Her disease and treatments made her feel tired. However, her work was important to her identity and she wanted to have the feeling of independence her work gave her for as long as possible:

> 'I find that if I'm working, I feel much better. I think it gives you a purpose. It takes your mind off the problems. I do feel I need to work you know.'

Johnson (1991) found that the process of regaining control after a heart attack involved three dimensions – an ability to predict outcomes, make informed decisions and act on decisions. The heart attack victims had a sense of uncertainty, which diminished predictability. They also had a lack of understanding of their bodies, undermining their sense of power and control. No longer able to trust their abilities and relying on others for support undermined their independence.

Some patients become excessively dependent on professionals or family members at an early stage of their terminal illness. They may be encouraged in this by their relatives or by the nurses caring for them and may be prevented from living as positively and fully as they might if they were more independent. Relatives can also become overdependent on staff, especially when the patient's terminal illness is a long one. They come to rely on certain staff members for support and this dependence can continue into bereavement. Occupational therapists are oriented towards encouraging patients to be as independent as possible, even in small ways, even when helping them would make things easier and quicker for the staff. It is not a kindness to encourage patients, even when terminally ill, to become too dependent, especially if there is a prospect of a remission or of their going home for a while. Decision making is an important part of autonomy. Doctors and nurses should encourage patients to be involved in treatment decisions.

Stigma

Having an advanced disease can be stigmatising and having advanced cancer especially so. Cancer victims may find that others do not accept them in the same way as before the diagnosis. In my research, cancer had frightening connotations for many patients (Lugton 1994). Edith felt that people would treat her differently because of her illness:

'People won't say that word, cancer. People have got visions of you sitting there fading away.'

Susan had had other illnesses but felt that having cancer was much more frightening:

'It was always referred to as the big C. It's a word that conjures up all different things in your mind. Cancer. I can't do this. I can't do that. I can't go there.'

We can promote a sense of belonging or social integration and not isolation in terminally ill patients by our own positive attitudes towards them, whether in hospital or in the community. People with advanced disease will feel reassured and valued if their families and friends spend time with them and accept them as 'normal'.

Sexuality

The threat to life posed by advanced disease does not always override anxieties about sexual identity. Sexuality is linked to self-concept, which, in turn, affects self-esteem and the ability to relate to others. In my research, support for sexual identity was as important for patients with advanced disease as for newly diagnosed patients (Lugton 1994). We should recognise that patients have to come to terms with feelings about body image and sexuality and be open to discussion of these topics with them.

Relationships

Important relationships may be impaired by illness. Lynam (1990) found that a cancer diagnosis was perceived by patients as threatening those relationships from which support was derived. Patients realised how threatening an illness could be to the people they cared about, as they too needed to confront the issue of mortality. All my respondents with breast cancer experienced some changes in their relationships during their illness (Lugton 1994). One man was initially unable to support his wife when she developed a recurrence:

> *'I think this kind of floored him. He couldn't come near me when I said "I've got to go for more tests". I just couldn't console him at all. I've always maintained that it's worse for the relatives. I always feel sad for the relatives who come into hospital when patients are maybe dying of cancer. I think there's an awful loneliness when they go away home. He appears to be fine now.'*

People need to be assured of the love of those closest to them and this need increases in times of crisis. Such attachments provide emotional support, esteem support and a sense of security. We can support patients' relationships by talking to relatives and finding out how they are coping.

Looking for cues

It is important to be sensitive to patients' verbal and non-verbal cues in order to assess their psychological needs and to offer appropriate support. Patients may indicate in a variety of ways that they want to talk to us about their illness, treatment or other problems. Of course, we too, consciously or unconsciously, give cues to patients and relatives about our own readiness to listen. We may sometimes recognise signs in ourselves, which indicate whether or not we are ready to enter into discussion with a patient. It is easy to forget that uniforms and hospitals can be intimidating and patients and relatives often rely on us to indicate that we have set time aside to talk to them.

In my hospice research, relatives were generally very satisfied with their communications with nurses, but a few relatives perceived areas of difficulty in initiating communication and obtaining the information needed, or support required

(Lugton 1987). Adequacy of communications was not linked to the length of the patient's stay. Sometimes a relative had visited the hospice for several days before he or she had spoken to a nurse apart from during the admission procedure. Some relatives seemed more willing to approach staff than others. Some admitted to being 'shy' while others felt that nurses should make the approach. A few relatives commented that they would have liked a member of the nursing staff to sit and talk to them and allow them opportunities for questions.

Potential problem areas

There are potential problem areas in breaking the news of a terminal illness or poor prognosis to patients and relatives, namely:

1 deciding who should tell
2 telling the relatives
3 explaining the meaning of symptoms
4 coordinating communications in the professional team
5 pacing disclosure of bad news
6 giving adequate follow-up support.

Deciding who should tell

The doctor is usually the person who discloses a terminal diagnosis to a patient and relatives. However, it may be the nurse who is available at the time that the patient plucks up the courage to ask about their illness. The nurse may be the person to whom the patient relates most easily, being involved in so much of their personal care. If medical and nursing colleagues work closely together, patients can be encouraged to seek information and express their anxieties without nurses becoming defensive in case they are asked awkward questions. Nurses who are prepared to listen to patients in such a way can help their medical colleagues to break bad news of a terminal diagnosis in a sensitive way. In some instances, when no doctor is available (e.g. at night), it might be kinder for the nurse to answer the patient's questions, rather than allow an opportunity to pass. If one member of staff is continually untactful when breaking bad news to patients, it is a clinical governance issue.

Telling the relatives

Despite recent moves towards more open disclosure of diagnosis and prognosis, it is still fairly common for the relatives to be given the diagnosis first and for the patient not to be told at all (Seale 1991, 1999). It has been argued that such deception, however well meant, denies the patient respect and may deny them the opportunity to take their proper leave of family and friends.

Sometimes a wife, husband, or other relative of the patient is told first of the terminal diagnosis. Implicit in this method of telling is the assumption that the patient will not be able to cope. However, apart from the ethical considerations of whether it is right to keep such information from the patient, there are dangers in this method. Patients and relatives may be unable to support each other because of the feeling that they must protect each other from the bad news. A conspiracy of silence can isolate family members at a time when they most need to trust each other. If the relative chooses not to tell the patient, this can leave the nurse in a very difficult situation, especially if the patient is obviously seeking more information. Sometimes a situation may arise where the relative knows about, and the patient suspects, the terminal illness, but neither is able to confide in the other. Children may also become caught up in the conspiracy of silence.

Opening up family communication is considered in more detail in Chapter 5, but at the time of diagnosis, patient and relatives should, if possible, be seen together by medical and nursing staff.

Explaining the meaning of symptoms

If no adequate explanation has been given about the meaning of symptoms, this may increase patients' fears. They may become concerned about new symptoms or the implications of an obvious deterioration in their condition.

Coordinating communications in the professional team

It is important for professionals to meet regularly as a team so that communication with, and support for, patients and relatives is planned. A record should be kept of important communications between doctors, nurses, patients and relatives about diagnosis, prognosis or treatment. If no such record is kept, it will be difficult to secure the maximum cooperation from professional colleagues in supporting patients and relatives. Patients will also be unable to trust a team whose members seem uncertain about their personal situation.

Pacing disclosure of bad news

The practice of most palliative care teams nowadays is to try to find out what the patient knows and to pace the disclosure (Buckman 1992). Breaking bad news about a terminal illness demands skills in listening, observation and empathy, as much as the ability to choose the right words. It is important to be aware of how much the dying person knows and how much they wish to know about their illness. There are no rules about when, how and what to tell, as each person must be treated individually. A team approach to talking with dying people is important, as each person should be able to seek information and help at the time they choose. The patient's confidence in the professional team will depend on all its members being sensitive and open in their communication with them.

Giving adequate follow-up support

Sometimes patients and relatives are told that a terminal illness has been diagnosed but thereafter are given little support by staff. General practitioners in the community may be unsure of what the patient has been told. As a result, communication can break down and valuable time is lost while decisions are delayed. When a terminally ill patient has been discharged from hospital, follow-up clinic appointments can cause more stress than benefit if it is obvious to the patient that the staff feel there is nothing more they can offer. If a district nurse or Macmillan nurse attends the clinic with the patient, he or she may be able to prompt the patient to ask about those things which are causing difficulties and thus make the visit worthwhile. Hospital nurses could do more to help such patients by taking time to explore with them any difficulties they are having at home, before they see the doctor.

Several studies have demonstrated the effectiveness of counselling in reducing stress in patients with cancer. For example, Maguire *et al.* (1980) found that where counselling occurred before and after operations for cancer of the breast, psychological distress was reduced.

Patients and relatives should be encouraged to ask questions and express their anxieties when a serious illness is suspected, when it has been diagnosed, and in the period following the diagnosis. Many of us will have had the experience of trying to help a relative or friend to cope with a serious illness and will be aware that he or she needed to talk to us often, about feelings and difficulties and treatment options. More nurses need to develop counselling skills to maximise the support that they can give to patients in the limited time available.

Questions and exercises

1 Which aspects of breaking news of a terminal illness or a poor prognosis to patients and relatives are most difficult for your team? Why is this so? How could you improve this situation?
   - Deciding who should tell.
   - Telling the relatives.
   - Explaining the meaning of symptoms.
   - Coordinating communications in the professional team.
   - Pacing disclosure.
   - Giving adequate follow up support.
2 In your experience, what important aspects of a person's identity or self-concept can be threatened by serious illness? How do you assess these threats? What support do you and your team provide?
3 As nurses we should aim to help people maintain and, if necessary, create their own informal support during illness. In what ways do you promote informal support from family, friends and other patients?

4

Assessing continuing needs for information and support

Breaking bad news should not be seen as a single event but a series of interactions over time. Sheldon (1993) noted that whether people express their needs depends on factors such as their expectations of treatment and their confidence in the ability of staff to help them. In my experience, the assessment of patients' and relatives' needs for information requires great sensitivity and skill from nurses, not only at the time of diagnosis, but in the following weeks or months of the terminal illness. As indicated in Chapter 3, awareness of a terminal illness does not always mean acceptance of its implications. Many people fear dying rather than death, imagining that they will have pain or other distressing symptoms and fearing that the doctors and nurses will be able to do little to help them. Relatives feel some degree of responsibility if a dying person is obviously suffering, and especially if they are caring for them at home. As nurses, we should help people to explore and express their anxieties so that we can give appropriate explanations and support. Nurses can usually give genuine reassurance that dying will not be as distressing as they may imagine. In my research, patients with breast cancer indicated that their coping ability increased with the availability of support from their health visitors (Lugton 1994). Health visitors' availability reduced patients' uncertainty. Patients looked to them for information and advice and health visitors enabled patients to cope better with psychological problems. Health visitors' support appeared to follow a counselling model and often incorporated the three aspects of Egan's (1990) helping model (this model is explored more fully in Chapter 9):

• Level 1 – The present scenario
• Level 2 – The preferred scenario
• Level 3 – Strategy: getting there.

One health visitor felt that some patients protected their doctors by not expressing their anxieties:

'Just listening was my main support for Jenny. A lot of patients feel that they can't tell the doctor how bad they feel because they feel that they are letting them down in a way.'

People who are terminally ill often have several distressing symptoms which may cause anxiety or embarrassment to themselves and their relatives. Symptoms such as dyspnoea or pain may be frightening, while incontinence or a fungating wound can be embarrassing. When staff take time to listen to such anxieties and to give explanations, much reassurance can be given. As one relative observed:

'The cancer went from the chest and lung up to the head. I visualised terrible things when it went to the head. The doctor explained what would happen. It made me feel better.'

It is important to try to find out how much patients and relatives wish to know about the illness or treatment so that information is given when requested and needed. Some people will want more information than others, and their needs will vary at different stages of the illness.

Understanding fears

A defined threat is usually less frightening because knowledge makes coping easier. Diagnosis of a terminal illness is stressful but can be less so than coping with uncertainty. Two of four areas of difficulty identified by Stedeford (1981) for terminally ill patients and their relatives, were coping with the direct effects of the illness and its treatment and inadequate communications both within the family and between patients, relatives and professionals. As Stedeford observed:

> *'Patients regarded general practitioners and hospital staff as erring on the side of saying far too little or else imparting information in an abrupt and blunt fashion.'*

The issue of whether or not to continue with treatment was raised by six couples in Stedeford's study, but the fear of uncontrolled pain was not a major concern because it was successfully controlled. Fears about insanity and loss of control were fairly common. Woodhall (1986) found that people's attitudes towards their illness and its symptoms seemed to be important in determining whether they stayed at home or were admitted to St Christopher's Hospice. Of home patients, 90% had mainly positive emotional responses to their illness in comparison with 63% of patients who were admitted to the hospice. This illustrates the importance of allowing people to express their anxieties and to receive emotional support at home.

Serious illness can have a devastating effect on people's emotions. Patients with advanced breast cancer worried about how long their disease could be controlled medically (Lugton 1994). In my hospice research (Lugton 1987), all the patients admitted to the hospice had undergone some physical deterioration prior to admission, and most had several distressing symptoms, with pain, immobility and/or falls being most frequently mentioned, followed by nausea/vomiting, dyspnoea and confusion. These symptoms were frightening for many patients and their effects are now examined in more detail.

Pain

†Where poorly controlled pain has been present, patients and relatives usually have distressing memories. Patients' experiences of pain should be explored and their anxieties respected, so that they are encouraged to report pain rather than suffer in silence. The following example illustrates the potentially devastating effects of uncontrolled pain.

> *'He's been ill for more than a year. He didn't get any strong painkillers at home. He was in agony, pain all the time. If he'd known what he was going to suffer, he'd have committed suicide. He couldn't get anywhere to put himself to be at rest.'*

Immobility and falls

Relatives often report their fear that a patient may fall. The fear of falls is a particular worry when the patient is living alone, or when an elderly relative is not strong enough to cope with the consequences of a fall.

'My Dad got so heavy and so difficult to move that my Mum just couldn't cope with him. She couldn't sleep having to be alert to his needs and she couldn't move him readily through to the toilet. She just cracked up. If he fell, she couldn't get him up again.'

Relatives' own assessment of how they are coping with the care of terminally ill patients should be explored and their perceived limitations respected.

Vomiting and nausea

It is worrying for relatives if a patient is unable to keep any food down, despite efforts to tempt him or her to eat. Also, constant nausea and vomiting leave a person feeling miserable. Patients and relatives need help on how to cope with this. They can be advised, for example, to serve small frequent snacks rather than large meals at set times. Examples 4.1 and 4.2 illustrate the problems patients and relatives can encounter.

Example 4.1

'In the last five or six weeks, it's been awful. The sickness hasn't eased. She really did deteriorate rapidly over the last few days. She felt so awful, she'd have gone anywhere, done anything.'

Example 4.2

'The main problem was the nausea all the time. She was sick during the night. If she saw a tray with a knife and fork, she'd be sick. My Mum's not been eating through the nausea and she couldn't take her anti-nausea medicine. That was coming up as well. It was like a vicious circle.'

Dyspnoea

Dyspnoea is perhaps the most frightening symptom for both patients and relatives. Often there seems little that relatives can do to help and their anxiety is conveyed to the patient, thus exacerbating the situation. Skilbeck *et al.* (1997) explored how nursing was delivered to individuals dying from chronic obstructive airways disease. Quality of life for these patients was poor and nursing skills were being under-utilised. The contact with community nurses was low and the main nursing input was in a hospital setting. Dyspnoea is particularly frightening for carers and patients to cope with at home. In Examples 4.3 and 4.4, relatives describe feeling helpless as the patient struggles for breath.

Example 4.3

'My husband's cough has been terrible. Talk about being frightened. It's as if he's going to choke. You can't do anything because you can't breathe for a person which is what you want.'

An elderly man was living alone and his son describes how his father would wake up at night, fighting for breath.

Example 4.4

'He was lonely, but he was more frightened because of his breathlessness. He would wake up at night and he had an attack. He couldn't breathe and there was nobody to help him.'

The perceived availability of medical and nursing staff seems to give many of these dyspnoeic patients a sense of security.

Skilbeck *et al.* (1997) found that three elements of nursing met the patients' needs; supportive care, monitoring and physical care. Supportive care included touch, verbal communication, and teaching patients to use breathing techniques.

Confusion

Confusion is difficult to cope with and sometimes causes acute embarrassment to relatives. It is considered in more detail in Chapter 5.

Expectations about treatment and symptom control

Patients and relatives feel more relaxed even when symptoms are not greatly alleviated, if nurses are perceived to be available and confident in their approach. The non-verbal reassurance patients and relatives can experience through the presence of experienced and attentive staff is as important as anything doctors or nurses may say to them. Hampe (1975) found that the patients' comfort was one of the most important factors in meeting relatives' needs.

In my own research, most relatives were satisfied that the patient was being kept comfortable and that symptoms had been alleviated, if not fully controlled. Patients' attitudes seemed to influence relatives' perceptions of the effectiveness of symptom control. If patients were content, the relatives were also happy with the level of care. Relatives' expectations of symptom control in the hospice were realistic, the major concerns being the comfort and contentment of the patient, rather than any dramatic improvement in his or her condition. One relative expressed the sentiments of many in this regard:

'I'm glad she's not suffering. She's comfortable. She's in people's hands who know what they are doing. She's getting her meals.'

Another relative recognised that her husband's condition was deteriorating, but was pleased that he seemed more comfortable and was able to enjoy his food again:

'Although he's gone down and down, I feel he's gone down and down in comfort, getting the medication right, the timing. He's eating more food here. He's enjoying his food. I think it's that he's with people who have got experience and that's what they want at this stage of their illness. They want to live as long as they can, so they want to know they're in the right hands.'

Sometimes relatives express a definite wish for palliative care in contrast to more active forms of treatment which they felt were no longer benefiting the patient. One relative felt that her mother's condition should not be subjected to further investigation:

'In hospital they said they were going to do body scans. I just wanted her here where she could get looked after properly.'

Relatives perceived some symptoms to be more successfully controlled than others, but most were alleviated to some degree. For example, pain was completely controlled or greatly alleviated in most cases and dyspnoea was alleviated in over half the cases. Several patients mentioned feeling secure although their symptoms had not always been completely controlled as Examples 4.5 and 4.6 show.

Example 4.5

'He knows if he coughs and gets into that terrible state, someone is there helping him. He knows he's safe.'

Example 4.6

'His biggest fear and worry was being on his own. He couldn't breathe. It's just the psychological effect here of knowing there's someone there to help him. He feels happy and he feels secure.'

Sometimes when symptoms are alleviated the patient or relatives seem almost to forget about the distress they caused.

'As far as I know, the vomiting has stopped and the pain has stopped too. She doesn't complain about them, so I presume they're not there.'

Assessment principles

The following factors will be important in assessing the needs of terminally ill people (Lugton 1999):

- establishing a relationship of trust with the patient and relatives
- identifying and classifying the patient's and relatives' needs
- prioritising the patient's and relatives' problems
- developing a multiprofessional approach to needs assessment
- making a diagnosis of nursing needs.

To be effective, assessment needs to be a two-way communication between nurses and patients so that patients can express their hopes and fears and receive information about their illness and its treatment. It is important not only to assess the severity of symptoms but also which of them troubles the patient most. A holistic approach implies multiprofessional involvement in the assessment.

Matching support to need

As nurses, we should be alert to situations where patients and relatives may be anxious and we should be prepared to give explanations about the effects of drugs the patient is receiving, procedures being carried out or about the appearance of new symptoms. In my research, patients and relatives seemed to want more information about the illness, symptoms or treatment when they were anxious about some aspects of these. Four relatives wanted to know more about the drugs the patient was receiving, and five about the effects of the illness. One patient had obviously been afraid of the implications of starting on morphine when at home. Examples 4.7 to 4.10 illustrate how easily misunderstandings can arise.

Example 4.7

'He was trying to conceal his pain from everyone. He was maybe trying to prolong the time before he started on morphine because, let's face it, when you start on morphine, you know you are critically ill. Everyone knows that morphine is for when you're critically ill, when you're very much in pain. I thought morphine was going to make him a bit dozy, but it didn't do anything to the brain. I had it wrong. They're still just as intelligent and alert.'

> **Example 4.8**
>
> 'I spoke to Dr Douglas because my sister was worried by the fact that she was dopey, so much under the influence of drugs. Dr Douglas said she would reduce the dose which I think she's done, without allowing the pain to intrude again.'

> **Example 4.9**
>
> 'I knew he was on diamorphine at home. I was worried about it, especially with a teenager at home. You can't have big bottles of diamorphine in the house.'

One man felt ambivalent about the prospect of his wife's discharge from the hospice because of his fears about a new symptom and how he could cope.

> **Example 4.10**
>
> 'She's got a new symptom now with this brachial plexus thing. I'm afraid of her becoming more paralysed. I hope it never happens. I think I'm going to have her home again. I don't know whether I'm strong enough. I wonder if it's even fair to expect that?'

Relatives' needs

Wright and Dyck (1984) explored the needs of cancer patients and their families. In this American study, the most frequently cited primary concerns related to dealing with symptoms, fear of the future, waiting and trying to obtain information. Relatives' highest priorities were to be kept informed of a patient's condition and to be assured that he or she was comfortable. Families of patients who were experiencing a recurrence of their cancer scored significantly higher on a 'need scale' than families at the time of initial diagnosis or during the terminal phase of the illness. Wright and Dyck (1984) comment:

> 'At this stage, families realise that the much hoped-for cure has not occurred and doctors and patients reach a communication impasse, thus isolating patients (and families) from the health care team and increasing their anxiety.'

Relatives had difficulty eliciting concrete answers from doctors, contacting doctors, getting information by telephone or finding out about the patient's daily progress from the nurses. Wright and Dyck comment on the prime position of nurses in easing emotional stress for patients and relatives:

> 'Families expect the nurses to explain daily procedures, treatments, medications and their possible side effects. This type of information is viewed as being helpful in terms of families being able to cope more realistically with the immediate future. The worry that accompanies waiting cannot always be eliminated.'

In my own research, most relatives did not want detailed information about drugs, treatment or the patient's illness if the patient seemed comfortable (Lugton 1987). This echoes Wright and Dyck's (1984) findings for relatives' needs in the terminal phase of a patient's illness. In a small study of patients with a terminal cancer diagnosis, Johnston and Abraham (2000) found that the amount of information sought from medical staff was sometimes limited by patients and relatives themselves rather than by staff. They did not want to be fully informed all of the time. In the hospice many relatives preferred to cope with their anxieties on a day-to-day basis, meeting difficulties as they arose. In Examples 4.11 and 4.12 two relatives explicitly mention feeling less need for information about the patient's illness and treatment than they did when they were in hospital because they knew that the illness was terminal, and also because they were confident that the patient would be kept comfortable.

Example 4.11

'I don't know what she's on. She's on injections every four hours, so I assume it's diamorphine. I know less than the staff know, but I know enough for myself. I know the state of affairs. If she were deteriorating a lot, they would ask to speak to me.'

Example 4.12

'I could speak to the doctors but they can't tell me any different from what I already know. I take it day by day. I use my own judgement when I see Jeanie.'

Hospital care

In McIntyre's research (1999) relatives of dying patients were critical of the poor amenities that hospitals provide for relatives' comfort and privacy, especially when relatives had to stay overnight in the wards. Relatives visiting dying patients in hospital often experience difficulties in knowing which nurse they should approach. Relatives were anxious not to be judged to be a nuisance and did not want to disturb a nurse who appeared to be busy.

Access to information

Relatives of dying patients consistently and repeatedly described their needs for information about the patient's care and progress and their need to have this information regularly updated (Lugton 1987, McIntyre 1999). The literature confirms that relatives appreciate information being offered to them, rather than actively having to seek it out. The family also appreciate having continuity of information and regular contact with the same member of staff. Relatives' information needs are not entirely straightforward – some days they want detailed information, at other times only the basic details about the patient's comfort.

McIntyre suggests that relatives be given some control over the timing, pace and volume of information to allow them to accommodate to their fluctuating capacity to confront the reality of their situation.

Helping relatives to cope

The stress that relatives experience is intensified when they feel unsure of what to expect and their information needs are not met. The hospital environment can be intimidating for relatives, and if the ward is made more welcoming and comfortable, this can enhance relatives' coping strategies. McIntyre (1999) found that relatives' stress was reduced when they could be with their loved one in a quiet, private setting and with access to facilities for rest and refreshment. Relationships between relatives and nurses were important and closer, more relaxed relationships between nurses and relatives yielded reciprocal coping benefits for both. Being in the relatives' role is hard work. Most relatives describe being exhausted, worn out or drained. They are likely to be sleeping badly and getting by on snacks rather than eating normally.

Giving sensitive support

Many writers have stressed the role of explanations and psychological support in alleviating patients' and relatives' anxieties about the effects of a terminal illness and its treatment. Such support is as essential as the medical treatment itself. It is easy for doctors and nurses to forget that patients and relatives may be worrying unnecessarily about the effects of drugs such as diamorphine, or that they may fear the imagined consequences of the spread of the disease to other parts of the body. It is equally easy for doctors and nurses to overlook the extent to which patients can naturally give support to each other, since they are often best placed to empathise with someone in a similar position to their own. Skilled support involves giving information when it is perceived to be needed by patients or relatives and being alert to situations when patients and relatives may be anxious. Too much information may provoke as much anxiety as too little, and it should always be tailored to the individual's needs.

In this chapter, I have explored some of the fears and anxieties of dying patents and their relatives. Their emotional responses to terminal illness can determine whether they live actively and positively, maintaining a hopeful outlook, or whether they are consumed by fear of what is happening to them or have anxieties about the future. The alleviation of physical distress does not depend exclusively on giving skilled physical care. It also depends on understanding and helping dying people with their fears. It is inevitable that patients and relatives will experience varying degrees of anxiety at the time a terminal illness is diagnosed, when there are signs of recurrence, or when it appears that a terminal phase has been reached. Our role should be to alleviate their fears by giving appropriate information and support and by the assurance that we will meet any problems together. Dying people and their relatives need to know that we are as interested and skilled in their palliative care as we were when there was a possibility of cure.

Questions and exercises

1 In what ways do you try to assess patients' and relatives' knowledge and anxieties about the symptoms or treatment of a terminal condition?
2 A holistic approach implies multiprofessional involvement in the assessment. How can this be achieved in your clinical area?
3 In McIntyre's research (1999), relatives of dying patients were critical of the poor amenities that hospitals provide for relatives' comfort and privacy. Is there anything that could be done to improve these amenities in your hospital?
4 How can relatives be better supported in the community?
5 Relatives are anxious not to be judged to be a nuisance and do not want to disturb nurses who appear to be busy. How do you ensure that this does not happen in your clinical area?

5

Planning support for family and close friends

Planning support

When a person with a potentially serious condition is being cared for in hospital, the needs of the family for information and support can often seem a lesser priority than making an early diagnosis and starting to treat the illness. Nurses are often in daily contact with relatives when they visit a person in hospital and are in a good position to be aware of their needs. In planning nursing support, it is important that the needs of the terminally ill person and their relatives and close friends are considered together. I have found that when family members are unable or afraid to share their feelings with each other much distress can arise. Relatives and patients can give each other mutual comfort and support if they are able to talk to each other openly and are not trying to protect each other by concealing their anxieties. I include children in the term relatives because they suffer when a loved parent or relative is ill, and can sometimes be excluded from the support professionals give to adult family members.

A number of authors describe as a journey the stages which family members go through when progressive illness strikes one of their members (Kristjanson and Ashcroft 1994, McIntyre 1996). This journey can start before the diagnosis is reached. In my research, I found that relatives and friends can undergo significant stress as their loved one undergoes a range of investigations (Lugton 1994). Joan's husband calmed her anxiety about clinic attendance:

'I went through all her staging with her. I went everywhere with her. Even when her biopsy was taken, she had to have me in the same room.'

Patients may see a large number of healthcare professionals making continuity of care and support difficult. Smith's (1996) research explored patients' recollections of their encounters with doctors during their cancer care. Interviews revealed that patients saw a large number of doctors. This appeared to confuse their medical management. Those who saw the same doctor at outpatient visits commented on the continuity of care they received.

During a progressive illness such as cancer, changes in family roles tend to take place and family members can encounter difficulties as they try to respond to subtle changes in the ill person's physical and emotional condition. This adaptation of family roles involves considerable hard work and negotiation often resulting in significant stress within the family. Families best able to adapt to these conditions have been found to be those where good communication had existed between the spouses before the onset of the illness and where the family included older children who could cope with expanded roles (Kristjanson and Ashcroft 1994). In my research, I found that most families accepted role changes induced by the patient's illness (Lugton 1994). Husbands were particularly helpful in this regard but sons, daughters and neighbours also offered practical help. Prior to her illness, Susan had normally done most of the housework despite having a demanding full-time job. However, her husband, son and daughter gave her a lot of practical help after her breast cancer diagnosis:

> *'The family have been absolutely wonderful. They managed quite well. In the past, I feel they've been dependent on me for lots of things. My daughter tries hard but she's a slow learner. She has stretched herself a bit more. Whatever she can do, she does.'*

Although many of these role changes were temporary, some were more lasting. Joan's husband was a workaholic, spending long hours in the family garage business. During her illness he promised to change:

> *'Sunday is family time. We've done lots of things that we should have done years ago, going for runs in the car, going out, taking the boys skiing and swimming and silly things like this. Life is too short. It's sad that it takes something like this to make you stop and take stock of things. It puts your priorities in place.'*

Maggie and her family appreciated each other more since her illness:

> *'I think I value my family more, particularly my husband. You begin to take them for granted and they take you for granted. That's not there any more. You plod along like every married couple does and when you face something like this, you realise how much you mean to one another again. We all say it, "What would we do if you weren't there? How would we cope as a family? What would we do with the kids? How would we tell the children?"'*

Individuals can experience their relationships as a mixture of support and strain. Patterns of support expectations are built up over time. However, people's social networks are not always capable of rendering support in a crisis. Family and friends may be unsupportive because their own needs are more pressing or because they feel personally threatened by the illness. When they become ill, some people have to seek new sources and types of support to complement what is provided by existing network members. In extreme circumstances they may have to weave entirely new networks. In my research, most unsupportive attitudes and behaviour towards the patient resulted from family, friends or neighbours being unable to cope with the patient's illness because of the perceived threat to their own identities (Lugton 1994). A terminal illness poses a threat to families' as well as to patients' futures, yet family members often receive less information and support from professional sources than do patients, although their anxiety may be almost as great. They may react negatively to disruptions in family routines and the threatened expectations that family members hold for one another as members of an interdependent system. In my research, the social networks of 14 families of women with breast cancer were predominantly supportive (Lugton 1994). Relationships among family members in this group seemed good. Nobody else had a serious illness to divert support away from the patient, and family and friends seemed able to cope with the patient's illness without perceiving it as threatening to themselves or to their position in the network. Janet had a large family who met frequently, communications were open and the sharing of problems encouraged:

'I've had great support from my family. My mother is still living and I've got four sisters. My daughter lives just round the corner. I see them all the time. I've got people round me if I want to speak to anybody about it. We are all very close. If I'm upset I would just phone one of them.'

The social networks of 18 families offered a mixture of support and strain. There were some longstanding relationship difficulties between women and their families in this group. In a number of cases, another person was ill or unable to cope with the woman's illness. Ellie, who had breast cancer, was trying to protect her husband who also suffered from ill health:

> 'I try not to say too much to my husband. Charlie, our younger son, came to the clinic with me. He is quite prepared. My husband is supportive to the degree that he keeps saying, "You are going to get better". I don't know whether that's just him hoping that I am.'

One patient suffered considerable strain from her family and her main support was her health visitor.

Identifying those needing support

As nurses, we should try to identify all the patient's family members, including children, at an early stage. Close friends of the patient should also be noted to ensure that no one is isolated from communication and support. This can happen when we communicate only with the next of kin. If one relative is being interviewed initially, we should ask if there are others with whom we should talk. A family tree diagram may be helpful in ensuring that a more complete picture is obtained (see Figure 5.1).

Family awareness and communication

There is evidence that relatives find communication with a dying family member extremely stressful (Seale, 1991). Participants in a study by Dunne and Sullivan (2000) described

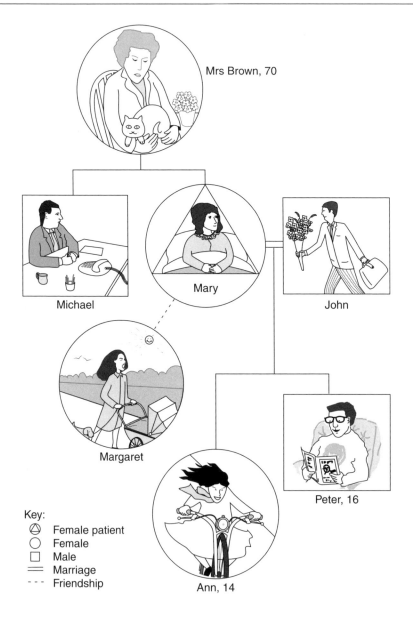

Figure 5.1   Identifying those needing support.

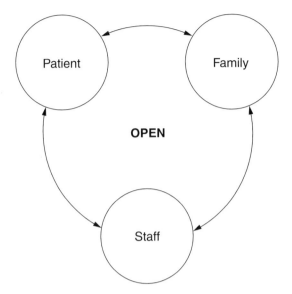

Figure 5.2   Open awareness and communication.

how difficult it was for them to communicate with their loved one in the period before his or her death. In their study, Glaser and Strauss (1965) noted that 'open awareness' and discussion of the terminal illness eased communication for staff, patient and family, while 'closed awareness' increased their difficulties. Open awareness is a situation in which each person feels free to discuss matters of concern with others (*see* Figure 5.2).

Where communication is 'closed', communication barriers exist. My hospice research revealed that interactions between patients and their relatives ranged along a continuum from completely open to closed (Lugton 1987). Confused patients and children were more difficult to place on this continuum.

Most relatives and patients were aware of the terminal nature of the patient's condition, but the extent to which this was discussed in the family varied. In seven families there were communication problems because the patient was confused or too ill to talk. In nine families communication between patient and relatives was poor for other reasons, e.g. the patient's anxiety and unwillingness to talk or patients' and relatives' desire to protect each other from painful awareness of the short time they would have together. We should not assume, therefore, that because both patients and relatives know the diagnosis, the implications of this knowledge have been discussed or that they have been able to share their feelings. Walter (1994) suggested that hospitals tend to be oriented more towards closed awareness patterns of communication, whereas hospices tend to adopt open awareness patterns in relation to patients knowing the truth about their terminal illness.

Open awareness

My research revealed that most families had discussed the diagnosis frankly and had considered the implications for the future of their surviving family members (Lugton 1987). Some relatives had taken on new roles since the patient's illness, for example, housekeeping or driving the car. It was very helpful to both patients and relatives to be able to discuss together their progress in coping with those changes.

Several patients and relatives had discussed the possibility of a relative moving house after the patient's death. A few patients and relatives had even discussed funeral arrangements. Three male patients had arranged their own funerals and one couple had discussed where the patient would be buried. The ability to talk together and express their feelings seemed helpful to both patients and relatives (Examples 5.1 and 5.2). One son said:

Example 5.1

'My dad's aware of what's wrong. We have no problems discussing things frankly. I mean, he wants to know. He said "You find out and tell me" and I've told him absolutely everything.'

Example 5.2

'We've talked the whole thing through, my wife and I. We spoke about the end. We said, "We've had a good life. We're 72. Aren't we lucky?"'

Closed awareness

Sometimes patients are unable to express their fears and anxieties about dying to their relatives. Relatives find this situation difficult and are often unsure of how to resolve matters, as Examples 5.3 and 5.4 show. The wife of one patient said:

Example 5.3

'I was speaking to Sister Alice. She said she thought he was a very frightened man which he is. He's been like this because they told him this would be his last winter. I've been frightened myself to approach him because I don't know how he's going to take it from me.'

One young man, recently bereaved, had wanted the hospice staff to help him talk to his father.

Example 5.4

'I'm sure he knew he had cancer, but it was something he never mentioned. I would have liked to have talked to him and perhaps even had a member of staff there for his own peace of mind. I think he knew he was dying anyway. I felt there was a barrier there. That's my one regret, that there wasn't enough talking.'

In fact, the hospice doctor had encouraged the patient and his wife to talk more openly to each other prior to hospice admission, but this openness had obviously not extended to the son.

Opening up communications within the family

Davies *et al.* (1994) noted that, in palliative care, the entire family is the focus of care but how nurses approach families depends on how the families are functioning. In families where there is open communication and flexibility in adapting to change, nurses can approach the family as a unit. In families where communication is indirect and where roles are rigidly defined, communication must be tailored to the family's level of functioning. Communications within the family may be helped if a nurse speaks to the family together, encouraging each member to express his or her feelings. Families use different methods to resolve their problems. Sometimes these are dealt with openly, or they may be only partly solved, leaving unresolved feelings. If there have been difficulties in relationships, there may be feelings of guilt, which need to be talked about openly. Sometimes conflicts cannot be resolved, but patients and relatives still need support. In every family, some role taking is inevitable, but sometimes roles are so fixed that change is difficult. It is important to talk to patients and relatives directly, either as individuals or as a family, as well as talking about them with colleagues. This will help to avoid 'labelling' patients and relatives as, for example, 'difficult', or reinforcing unhelpful patterns of interaction within the family. In my research, patients with breast cancer sometimes felt able to discuss with health visitors, concerns that they felt unable to mention to families or friends (Lugton 1994).

> *'That's what you need sometimes, someone to be an outsider coming in that you can bounce things off. I think it's quite*

normal when you've got a family. You've got to put this façade on. You don't want to upset them. It's safe to talk to her (health visitor) about private things, confidentially.'

The patients' and relatives' pace in coming to terms with their situation has to be respected by staff who are giving support, and it should be recognised that patients and relatives may be at different stages in their grieving. Relatives and patients expect, rightly, that while open and honest communication will be encouraged, this will be done in a sensitive way.

In my research, one elderly couple had been very anxious when the husband was a home-care patient. On admission, a hospice doctor encouraged more open communication between them by talking to them together (Lugton 1987). The patient's wife describes this meeting.

'The doctor said: "Do you ever talk to your husband about these things?" I said, "Well, sometimes I do". He said, "I want you to tell your husband everything. You're both married. You both know all about each other. You're worried about him. He's worrying about you. If there's anything at all, you speak to your husband about it and your husband will speak to you. You'll get relief by talking about it". It's true. It helps, because we were frightened to say anything to each other at first.'

Obviously, acceptance of a harsh reality is more difficult for some people than for others. A few relatives openly express a wish not to be told about a patient's prognosis and prefer to take each day as it comes.

Confused patients

Relatives often have difficulties in communicating with confused patients. Confusion sometimes causes embarrassment to relatives who find it difficult to relate to someone with whom they can no longer communicate. One hospice patient had a brain tumour and his wife had been embarrassed on several occasions by his behaviour whilst at home (Example 5.5).

> **Example 5.5**
>
> 'He was hyperactive. He was getting lost and being brought back by the police. His mental condition went down. He couldn't eat properly, see properly. His memory was so bad. We had one or two outbursts when we were at the shops.'

The daughter of the man described above was very upset because in her last conversation with him, her father had told her to 'Go away'. Shortly after his admission to the hospice, he became unconscious, so she felt that she had been unable to say good-bye to him. Some confused patients have little insight into what is happening to them (Example 5.6).

> **Example 5.6**
>
> 'She has been told. It seems to be a mental block. Not long ago, when she was beginning to get really bad, she said, "What was it the doctor said was wrong with me?" She's a bit confused and there's lots of things she isn't taking in.'

A young woman worried about how nurses would react to her mother who was a little confused and seemed unhappy (Example 5.7).

> **Example 5.7**
>
> 'I think the staff are seeing her as not a very nice person, whereas I know that in her true self, she's not really like she is now. I feel that

makes them not like her as much as I would like them to like her. I spoke to one of the staff nurses. She was very concerned and she was well aware that she's not always been like that.'

Supporting relatives of confused patients

Developing understanding in the care of the confused patient is important, since it is often the relatives who suffer most in this situation. We can help relatives with the stigma of having a family member who is confused by demonstrating that the person has not lost all dignity or right to respect and by trying to learn from the relatives what the person was like before he or she became confused. Stedeford (1981) found that mildly confused patients responded with great relief to reassurance such as 'Whatever odd things your brain tumour makes you say or do, I still know that you, yourself, are all right'. This enabled people to distinguish between concepts of 'myself' and 'my illness'.

Clear signals can keep confused people orientated towards reality. For instance, good lighting, a clock at the bedside, siting the bed near the toilet or near the window and having a daily routine, are all helpful, especially when the person is in unfamiliar surroundings. We should encourage confused patients to talk about their fears which may sometimes aggravate confusion, and show relatives the value of non-verbal communication in showing love and concern to the confused person. Sometimes in hospital, relatives are afraid to touch the patient or to take the 'cot sides' down unless they are encouraged to do so. Familiar items such as family photographs may encourage the confused person to remember important family events, and also give relatives the opportunity to talk to staff about the patient's past life, thus removing some of the stigma of confusion and revealing the 'real' person behind the present condition. Sometimes the confused person's memory for past events is quite good, even when the short-term memory is poor. The relative quoted earlier whose husband had a cerebral tumour, commented on his obvious enjoyment of visits to the day hospice despite his failing memory.

> *'He had three visits to the day centre. He'd met other people and he's met someone who had been in India sometime and had a chinwag because he remembered things from long ago. But even things from long ago are getting a bit muddled up.'*

Communicating with children

Children need particularly sensitive understanding to help them cope with impending bereavement, and their awareness of the terminal illness and needs for support should be explored and determined. Raphael (1984) noted that a child's response to death should be viewed in a family context. Parental attitudes to death, openness with children and the support they receive from the extended family can be an important influence on children's attitudes. In my own research (Lugton 1987), communication between adult family members and children seemed to be fairly open, possibly because most children in my study were losing a grandparent and not a parent. Experience at St Columba's Hospice has shown that problems may arise in their bereavement if children are not involved when a close relative is terminally ill.

The serious illness of a parent may threaten the security of children. In my research with women who were being treated for breast cancer, some school-age children developed behaviour problems at school or at home (Lugton 1994). Harriet's son, aged 15, had to cope with his father's illness (subarachnoid haemorrhage) as well as his mother's breast cancer:

'He went away when I was in hospital to stay with my cousin who he is very fond of because he couldn't hack it anymore he said. I know it's affected his schoolwork. He's lost a lot of self-confidence but the school is aware of why.'

Very young children and babies will not necessarily fully understand but will be aware of a dramatic situation. They may not have the words to express what they are feeling but they must be told what is going on. They need more attention and explanation than usual. In the hospice, difficulties in coping with a parent's or grandparent's terminal illness are not always related to age, as older children are sometimes more withdrawn and uncommunicative than their younger siblings. Examples 5.8 to 5.10 illustrate this point:

A four-year-old girl knew that her mother was going to die and wanted to talk about it to her father.

Example 5.8

'Ann knows her mum's dying. She said "Mummy's going to God, isn't she?" I said, "Yes". She's only four and a half. It's no use telling the bairn lies, saying her mum will be away and she'll be back. I'm just preparing her in a nice way. She'll never forget her mother, but she's young. She's got her own life to lead.'

Example 5.9

'My own kids have seen him throughout. I think my son may be reacting in some way. He's twelve and my daughter's nine. My son doesn't say terribly much. My wife was talking to him and my son was saying he didn't know what to say to grandpa. There have been too many other people there. We've talked to them about the whole thing.'

One teenager was afraid of being in the house when her grandmother died.

Example 5.10

'My youngest daughter (16) was frightened of her grandmother dying in the house. She said, "If anyone died in this house, I would have to move". Before my mother got too bad, she was in the house with her. She was off school. She said, "I'm frightened nanny dies when I'm here". I've said to her "That isn't likely to happen because with the illness she's got, they gradually get worse and you know a long time beforehand".'

Visiting

Sometimes children are discouraged from visiting because relatives feel that it would be a strain or an embarrassment for the dying patient or because they feel that the children could be upset by what they may see. Patients' attitudes to children's visits are also important. A few hospice patients do not want their children or grandchildren to visit them when their condition deteriorates. While patients' and relatives' wishes must be respected, they may appreciate an opportunity to discuss their feelings with a nurse. For example, one boy was helped to cope with his father's impending death by witnessing the peaceful death of another patient on the ward.

Supporting children

We should take time to speak to children and teenagers individually, as well as to adult family members. As with adults, it would be helpful for one or two nurses to introduce themselves by name. There are occasions when parents would appreciate the opportunity to talk to nurses about a child who is withdrawn or seems anxious, or to seek advice about whether a child should continue to visit when the patient's condition deteriorates.

In St Columba's Hospice, several relatives wanted to talk to staff about what to say to children. This is a sensitive area, but nurses may be able to support younger children by just talking to their parents or grandparents and encouraging openness within the family. Teenagers in particular may appreciate talking to a nurse or doctor alone. Facilities such as a coffee lounge, a play area, or crèche may help children to feel more at home when visiting a relative in hospital. Fostering an attitude among nursing staff that recognises the distinctive relationships that exist between each member of the family and the patient, should be a key objective of the nursing approach.

In this chapter I have tried to show that the needs of dying people and their relatives are interrelated. We should be aware of all family members and close friends of each patient and of any difficulties they may be experiencing in talking openly to each other. It may be helpful, on occasions, to talk to the patient and relatives together, encouraging them to share any anxieties and perhaps to demonstrate more explicitly their concern for each other. It should not be assumed that the preparation of children for bereavement should always be left to the parents and grandparents, or that this is what the latter would wish. In my experience, families of terminally ill patients are often very grateful for the assistance of a professional person, doctor or nurse who understands that they have needs distinct from those of the patient and who does not make them feel selfish in expressing those needs.

Questions and exercises

1 What steps do you take to identify all close relatives and friends of a terminally ill patient who may need support?

2 Do you try to identify the principal carer? In what ways can you give additional emotional support to the principal carer?

3 A case is quoted in this chapter where a son wanted a nurse's help in opening up communication between him and his father. How would you have tried to help them?

4 How do you support children and adolescents who are relatives of a dying person? What do you do well? What aspects of your support could be improved?

5 Are you usually aware when communication barriers exist within families? How do you identify these barriers? When they seem too strong to be broken down, how then should the situation be managed?

6 The stages which family members go through when progressive illness strikes one of their members have been described as a journey. How do you support the family in the earlier as well as the later stages of the journey?

7 A terminal illness poses a threat to families' as well as to patients' futures. How can you ensure that families receive the information and support they need?

6

Preparing relatives for bereavement

Relatives' preparation for bereavement begins in the preceding weeks or months of the person's terminal illness and not at the time of death. This period of preparation also provides an opportunity for nursing staff to support and counsel relatives. We can encourage them to express feelings and fears and keep them fully informed of any changes in the patient's condition. There may be opportunities to encourage family members to be more open with each other and to listen to their anxieties about the future.

In a sense, everything that is done for the patient and relatives prior to death is part of the preparation for bereavement. Relatives will probably remember any special consideration shown to them by staff and whether the person was comfortable and peaceful in the last days. On the other hand, any perceived neglect on the part of staff will also be remembered and perhaps magnified beyond its original significance.

Worden (1991) describes four tasks which mourning seems

to fulfil:

1 to accept the reality of the loss
2 to experience the pain of grief
3 to adjust to an environment in which the deceased is missing
4 to relocate the dead person internally (*see* p.97).

The ways in which people may be helped in the first three of these tasks are now considered.

Accepting the reality of impending loss

In St Columba's Hospice, most relatives are fully aware of the terminal nature of the person's illness, but their degree of acceptance of the impending loss varies. Some relatives do not fully accept the implication of terminal illness, although they are aware of the diagnosis.

> *'I spent my time keeping my spirits high and refusing to listen to people. I felt I was fighting them by always sounding hopeful, but we'd had so many disappointments. I've read all the literature and wept for miracles. All this time I've been indulging in prayer and all kinds of healing things and applying my strength to telling this ruddy thing to push off.'*

It is helpful if the relatives' and patient's awareness of the diagnosis is marked in the case notes. Understanding is, however, at two levels, intellectual and emotional. Relatives who are aware of the diagnosis may not accept all its implications, for example the prognosis or the advent of new symptoms. These should be pointed out gently to them by staff as each problem arises or change occurs. In my experience, most relatives do not wish to look too far ahead and prefer to ask for and receive information on a day-to-day basis. In trying to accept their impending bereavement, many relatives become anxious and some express extreme anxiety as the following example illustrates:

'I'm just terrified. I know my husband used to go away when he was at sea, but I knew he was there. I could always talk to him when he came home. I don't know how I'll cope. I was sitting in the coffee lounge and I felt I just couldn't move. I felt as if I was rooted to the spot. I knew I'd got to get home but I couldn't get a bus. I ordered a taxi in the end.'

Sometimes, very anxious relatives are helped to cope with their anxiety by involvement in the patient's nursing care. There are many simple tasks which they can easily perform – washing, feeding and combing the patient's hair. Relatives may benefit from such involvement so long as they feel the decision to act in this way is theirs. Home commitments, fatigue, and the wishes of the patient may mean that some relatives do not or cannot become very involved in even simple nursing.

Experiencing the pain of grief

In my hospice research, most relatives had begun to think of the future without the dying person and some had begun to make some sort of plans. Several relatives talked about feelings of loneliness. Many relatives wanted to express their feelings and talk about family problems or other difficulties they had faced or were still experiencing. Hampe (1975) found that relatives of terminally ill people needed opportunities to ventilate their own emotions and to receive support from family members and health professionals. We should, therefore, plan our support of relatives so that we make a point of letting them know that we care about these anxieties and that we understand their feelings. If possible, they should be taken somewhere private and be given the opportunity to talk and ask questions of however simple a nature. If relatives successfully try to suppress their feelings too much, family and professionals can assume all too easily that they are coping well and do not need further support. This can give rise to real difficulties as shown in the following quotation from an elderly man:

> 'It's something I've never done before is wept at anything, but I'm afraid this has been a bit of a shaker. The tears come so easily and I feel so stupid about it, you know. My own doctor said "You can let it come because you've held it in too long". I said, "I've never cracked before". This is something which in our generation they didn't do. I believe they do it more now. It's a release you know.'

When a patient dies in a hospice, a nurse usually spends a little time talking to bereaved relatives about the formalities of registering the death and about funeral arrangements. There is also an opportunity to comfort the relatives and to talk about how they are feeling or may feel in the future.

One young man, who had been bereaved when his father died in the hospice, had found his talk with a hospice sister very helpful:

> 'The help before and after my father's death was very good. The fact that the sister took my sister and me through to one of the rooms and had a nice chat to us. It calmed us down for the trauma of going home and trying to explain it to the rest of the family.'

When encouraging relatives to talk about their future, we can discourage them from making hasty decisions based on their present feelings and which they might later regret. For example, some relatives consider moving house because their home is too big or has too many memories of their loved one. They may not have explored the implications of moving away from friends and neighbours whom they have known for years and who would be well placed to give them support. Many bereaved people will be living alone for the first time. In my hospice research (Lugton 1987), most seemed well supported by family and friends; seven relatives were considering moving house and five of those were living alone. An elderly man interviewed during bereavement was concerned about his sister who was living alone:

> 'She left her sister very comfortable in a lovely home, but I think we may get her down beside us. She'd be better down beside us.'

A relative of another patient had been ill herself:

> 'I can't stay on my own. I will go south to my son. I did wonder about staying here on my own but I can't. I never know when I'll be paralytic with chest pain.'

One woman was going to discuss her options with friends who had themselves been bereaved:

> 'In the first place, I'm doing nothing for a while, but I think I'll have to get a smaller flat because this house has four bedrooms. What I would like is to see friends around the country and stay with them, one or two widows and discuss it with them and see what they did and then decide where to live.'

One elderly man rejected the idea of living with his son after his wife's death:

> *'I've looked at everything fairly carefully during this period when my wife's been told it was terminal. I've thought things through fairly well. I'm still living at home and I have my meals with my son, but I prefer to go home to my own bed. I'll just have to adjust, you see. I have a garden. I'm one of those fortunate people whose work was his hobby. Apart from the war years, I've worked in gardens all my life.'*

Where new roles have to be learned, it can be a great help to both patient and relatives if a beginning is made before the patient dies. Some male relatives, for example, have to learn to cook and do their own housework for the first time. Female relatives may have to learn how to cope with financial matters or learn to drive. A few people may fail to adapt or patients may resent partners taking on roles they had previously enjoyed. It is helpful for relatives to discuss and rehearse how they might cope with radical changes in life-style. One elderly man had been talking to his terminally ill wife in the hospice about his management of the house-keeping and had been helped by her encouragement and that of his sister-in-law:

> *'It's very quiet in the house just now, on my own. I just couldn't understand what had happened to me, walking into an empty house and starting to do things for myself. We've no family and we're more or less always together. I was very, very shocked. Mattie's a bit more settled now. Her sister has been up and said, "He's doing fairly well in the house. He's got it in good condition". That cheers her up.'*

It is not only learning new roles that is difficult, but adapting to the loss of close companionship, shared ideas, interests, humour and even disagreements.

Adjusting to an environment in which the dying person is missing

Many people have begun to cope alone while their relative is still alive because they recognise the need to take on new roles and responsibilities. This is true not only for relatives of cancer patients but for families of people with longer-term illnesses such as strokes and motor neurone disease. We should talk to relatives about these changes and how they feel they are going to cope, and honestly explore their capacity to cope. If relatives are helped to explore their plans for the future, even if only tentatively, their options may become clearer to them and possible consequences come to light which had not been considered previously. It may sometimes be easier for relatives to discuss future plans with an outsider, rather than a family member who might pressurise them into making particular decisions, which might not be their wish.

Relocating the dead person internally

Worden (1991) amended his fourth task of mourning from 'withdrawing emotional energy and investing it in another relationship' to 'relocating the dead person internally'. Thus he strongly suggests that a continued relationship with the dead person is both appropriate and necessary. Stroebe *et al.* (1993a) also note the importance of an ongoing relationship with the deceased person. This may involve, for example, visiting places or participating in activities that both the bereaved and the dead person enjoyed, keeping memories alive through photographs and 'talking' to the dead person. Walter (1996) suggests that those who are bereaved may benefit from talking about the deceased person with others who knew the person. Through such conversations, the bereaved person is able to integrate memories of the dead person. Walter suggests that bereaved people need to make sense of their experiences through 'progressive, reflexive narrative which enables the relocation of the dead person in the memory'. We can encourage them to reflect on their memories as the hospice sister did in the following example:

> *'I can't remember all of it, because I think my brain was put into neutral. Certainly the sister, I think, had gone through the experience. She was saying "You'll have the up days and the down days and it'll suddenly hit you sometimes if you see a photograph or if you're going through clothes or something. It'll spark off a memory". I find it difficult to visualise my father in his last days. I can only remember the good days. So her experience was true for myself.'*

The son, in the case quoted above, had few distressing or negative memories of his father. It is important to remember that people who have ambivalent relationships often have difficulties in bereavement. However, nurses may need to help people express their negative feelings of anger, guilt and resentment, as well as those of sorrow, loss and gratitude, by their own accepting and non-judgemental approach. Talking to relatives about the experience of bereavement and how they may feel at this time may help them to cope with the low points later on in their bereavement.

Identifying relatives needing extra support

Some people experience pathological grief which leads to lasting problems. It is important to target bereavement interventions towards these people. There has been a great deal of research into risk factors. Risk factors are now considered in more detail. They have implications for support of relatives during the person's terminal illness and their own bereavement.

Unexpected loss

While unexpected loss does increase vulnerability, prolonged dying can also heighten the risk of grief problems (Stroebe *et al.* 1993b).

Self-esteem

Variables such as positive self-esteem and personal competency in coping with everyday life are predictive of a better bereavement outcome (Lund *et al.* 1993).

Dependent or ambivalent relationships

Raphael (1984) noted that certain groups of people seemed more at risk of having difficulties during bereavement. She identified those with close, dependent or ambivalent relationships as being 'at risk'. In my hospice research, several future widowers had close, mutually-dependent relationships with their wives in the sense that they were always together and seemed to have few close relationships outside marriage. In other instances, long-standing marital problems may present difficulties to the surviving person during bereavement. Where difficulties in relationships are long-standing, positions have often become entrenched and difficult to change. Help may best be given by not taking sides and by pointing to the positive features in the relationship, past or present, whenever possible. We may be able to encourage family members to act differently in small ways and this may help the relationship overall. For example, we could encourage a husband to show affection to his wife more openly, by telling her, perhaps for the first time, that he appreciates all she has done for him. If we have endeavoured to listen to the patient and various individual relatives, there will be less temptation to label particular people as 'difficult'. Where there are disputes in the family about who should visit and when, the patient's wishes should be noted and respected.

Concurrent stresses

Raphael (1984) noted that those undergoing a concurrent stress at the time of bereavement were more at risk of a difficult bereavement. Sometimes relatives have to cope with more than one sick person in the family, or a recent bereavement as well as the impending death of the patient. Such people will need particular understanding if they are to cope with the compounded stress such situations produce.

Low perceived support

Research has shown that a perceived low level of support is a risk factor in bereavement. Perceived support is often more important than actual support in determining the outcome of a bereavement. People who perceive themselves as being unsupported, may be unable to accept support when it is offered. In my hospice research, most relatives seemed well supported, but a few perceived themselves as not having much support. These were mainly people who had had long and close marriages. Single people and close friends may be overlooked when assessing support. For example, an unmarried daughter may have been living with an elderly parent for many years and may have lost many of her own social contacts with her parent's increasing dependence. Unmarried sisters and brothers may have spent a lifetime together. For these people, the dying person may be as much at the centre of their existence as a husband or wife. There may be a long period after the person's death when they will feel intense loneliness. They may be helped, however, by the gentle and unobtrusive support of friends and relatives. If we are aware of such friends and relatives, we may be able to suggest to them ways in which they could make their support more effective. We can stress the helpfulness of a sympathetic, listening ear and of acceptance of the importance of their loss. Practical help with shopping and preparation of meals may be important for elderly people. The bereaved person may have become socially isolated and need to develop social contacts with both sexes.

Other avenues of support should be explored with a view to the future, since the relative may not feel able to accept them immediately after the person's death, e.g. church connections, lunch clubs and home help services. Spiritual help may give great comfort to some relatives. A word with the chaplain or clergyman about funeral arrangements is usually helpful. Relatives who have no church connections may fear an impersonal funeral where the minister or priest knows neither the patient nor the family.

Children

When a person dies, the adult relatives are sometimes so absorbed in their own grief that children in the family who are also grieving do not get much opportunity to express their feelings. Liaison with the child's school is important so that teachers are aware of the reason for behaviour changes and can be supportive rather than critical. Community nurses can assist in this. In my research with patients with breast cancer, health visitors spoke to patients' children to find out how they were coping (Lugton 1994). In some areas, counsellors from the bereavement organisation, CRUSE, work with bereaved children in the schools. The teachers have referred these children to the counsellors because of the onset of behaviour problems since their bereavement.

Wright (1996) facilitates a clinic for suddenly bereaved children. He described possible responses of children to the news of a sudden death as follows:

- shock and disbelief
- dismay and protest
- apathy, withdrawal
- continuation with usual activities.

Children's age and understanding of death

Children's understanding of death varies with age but honest explanations and allowing children to talk about their feelings are important regardless of age. Younger children may be unable to understand the permanence of death and may think that a parent, who has died, will return. Jobling (1975), summarising research findings into bereavement among children, wrote:

> *'Very young children have limited comprehension but seeing death as separation, may react with profound grief. While pre-school children may be bewildered or may appear callously to ignore death, this is a time when parents are most needed as identification models ... Five to eight year olds are in the stage of "magical thinking", believing that wishing can make something come true ... They often become especially good and conscientious, as if in hope of restoring the dead. At about nine, children express sorrow as adults do – they may be apathetic, withdrawn, cry a great deal or become hostile and angry.'*

Wright (1996) found that the age of a child can affect his or her perception of death. Children under five years old lack understanding of the finality of death, those under ten years old had a more 'literal understanding' of death, while those over ten years had a more abstract understanding, and were likely to have strong emotional reactions. He noted that boys may be given messages about being strong and in control while girls could more overtly express their grief.

Bereavement and people with learning disabilities

As nurses we may not always adequately consider the needs of people with learning disabilities who suffer bereavement. Some of the difficulties of supporting people with learning disabilities are illustrated in the following example. A patient admitted to St Columba's Hospice had a son with Down's syndrome in hospital and had been visiting him faithfully three times a week before she became ill. Her daughter was going to take over this responsibility from her mother but had found it impossible to explain to him about his mother's illness. She said:

> '*I have a young brother in hospital. He's handicapped and he doesn't speak. He's quite low grade so I can't even explain to him about her. It's quite sad really. Mum's stopped speaking about him. I don't know if it's all going over her head now or whether she realises she can't go now anyway.*'

Several studies maintain that the concept of death in adults with learning disabilities resembles the concept of death in children. Other authors are reluctant to view age as the sole determinant of understanding illness and death. Bihm and Elliot (1982) suggested that the development of the concept of death in people with learning disabilities was related to their cognitive level rather than their age. Cathcart (1995) points out that, as in the general population, bereavement outcome in people with learning disabilities is likely to depend on many factors such as gender, social support, the nature of the relationship and the manner of the death.

How can we better support people with learning disabilities during bereavement? Strachan (1981) studied bereavement reactions among adult residents with learning disabilities and found that, for long-term residents, more marked responses were often reported by nurses to deaths of other residents on the ward than for those of close relatives. Few of the residents were able to maintain contact in the terminal stages of their relative's illness, with news of the death being broken in most cases by ward staff after they had been informed by telephone. Strachan recommends that ward staff should arrange a visit to the sick relative at home, hospital or hospice and that, whenever possible, a family member should break the news to a hospital resident. The handicapped person's need to participate in the funeral may be important even if understanding is limited. Cathcart (1991) suggested making up a personal album about the relationship with the dead person which incorporated 'photos, drawings or illustrations from magazines. It could also include a piece of familiar clothing, which may have comforting associations of touch and smell'. There are three short books about death and people with learning disabilities entitled *Understanding Death and Dying* (Cathcart 1994). The first book in the series is for clients, the second for families supporting a friend or relative with learning disabilities and the third is for professionals and other carers.

Bereavement follow up

Some palliative care teams have meetings to try to identify relatives who might be having a difficult bereavement and who need extra support. Such an assessment is subjective and is made by doctors and nurses and sometimes other team members who knew the bereaved relative either at home or at the hospice. General practitioners are notified if the team feels concerned about a particular relative. The relative could, if he or she wished, be put in touch with CRUSE, a national organisation for the bereaved. There are now a number of other support groups for the bereaved, e.g. The Stillbirth and Neonatal Death Society (SANDS) and The Compassionate Friends. The latter organisation is for parents who have lost a child. Society, as well as individuals, is developing expertise in supporting the bereaved in other traumatic situations, e.g. after the Bradford football stadium fire.

It is possible, even during a short interview with relatives, to elicit important factors which may affect bereavement outcome. We should be aware that time spent talking to relatives and exploring these areas is likely to lead to a more accurate assessment of relatives' needs for support from us during the terminal illness and from professional colleagues and voluntary organisations during bereavement. Parkes and Weiss (1983) and Levy *et al.* (1992) noted that nurses' judgement of the person's ability to cope had a high predictive value. Walshe (1997) therefore advocates that risk assessment tools, designed to enhance the identification of those who could benefit from bereavement intervention, should not replace clinical, holistic nursing assessment. They should be used to add a degree of objectivity to the assessment.

In this chapter, I have tried to show how much can be done to prepare relatives for bereavement during the person's terminal illness as well as at the time of death. Just as the dying person may experience different phases in coming to terms with their illness, so their relatives and close friends begin a grieving process which will continue into bereavement. There are many opportunities to help relatives in these 'tasks of mourning'. If we are also aware of those relatives who may be 'at risk' during bereavement, we can offer them extra support ourselves by putting them in touch with professional colleagues or with a voluntary organisation such as CRUSE which specialises in meeting their needs.

Questions and exercises

1 How do you help relatives to prepare for bereavement? Do you help them in any of the ways mentioned in this chapter? i.e.:
   • Helping them towards acceptance of the terminal diagnosis and prognosis.
   • Encouraging them to recognise and express their emotions.
   • Suggesting practical ways of helping them to adjust to changes in lifestyle, role, etc.
   Add your own suggestions, based on your own experience.
2 How do you support relatives at the time of a patient's death? Do you discuss any of the following matters with them?
   • What has been written on the death certificate?
   • Registering the death and funeral arrangements.
   • Their own feelings at the time of death.
   • How they may feel during bereavement.
   • A commitment to counselling support if they wish it.
3 Do you use any information leaflets in supporting bereaved relatives? In what ways might such leaflets be useful? Suggest some improvements to the material you have used in the past.
4 It is possible, even during a short interview with relatives, to elicit important factors which may affect bereavement outcome. How do you identify relatives in need of extra support from you and your colleagues both during the terminal illness and during bereavement?
5 What arrangements, if any, do you make for follow-up of the bereaved either by yourself or others?
6 How can you better support people with learning disabilities during bereavement?

7

Making communication more effective

In our personal lives, we are aware that our most meaningful communications take place in the context of warm and trusting relationships. As nurses, we should try, therefore, to relate to dying people and their relatives on a personal as well as a professional level. Thompson *et al.* (1983) described the relationships which can develop between dying people and professional carers as 'covenant' relationships, in contrast to the code and contract relationships more appropriate in other situations.* Carers are at the limit of what they can do in a curative sense and they offer the patient palliative care, support and befriending. By encouraging dying people to be involved in decisions about their own care and treatment

*When a relationship is governed by contract, the person in need can make his or her own decisions, and can seek help elsewhere. Both the carer and the person in need have contractual rights and duties towards one another. When a relationship is governed by code, the carers have to decide what is in the best interests of the person in their care because the person is unable to make decisions for himself.

whenever possible, they ensure that those aspects of care which enhance quality of life receive priority.

Nursing theory now stresses the importance of a person rather than a task-oriented approach to patients and their relatives. An essential part of individualised care for the dying is good communication between patient, relatives and staff. Heaven and Maguire (1996) recommended that communication skills courses should include input on the handling of emotions and that courses need to challenge nurses' attitudes and beliefs about their skills and examine the consequences of their actions on patients. Bailey and Wilkinson (1998) conducted a pilot study to ascertain patients' views of nursing communication skills and to examine their experience of an assessment interview. The assessment interview aimed to facilitate patients to discuss their illness and concerns. The study involved registered nurses who had completed a university course in cancer or palliative care. The aim was to find out whether nurses' communication skills had been retained over time (four years since their completion of the course). Thirty-six patients with advanced cancer were invited to participate. Twenty-nine patients returned their questionnaires. Twenty-seven patients were very satisfied and two were fairly satisfied with their interaction with the nurse. Eighty-six percent said that they had no other concerns that they would have liked to have discussed with the nurse. Four patients mentioned additional concerns that they would have liked to have discussed with the nurse. Wilkinson *et al.* (1998) found a significant improvement in the depth and breadth of the assessment interviews, especially in emotionally-laden areas such as patients' awareness of their diagnosis.

Non-verbal communication

Although verbal communication is an important channel of support, there are other powerful, but less well recognised, dimensions. It is important to be sensitive to patients' verbal and non-verbal cues in order to assess their psychological needs and to offer appropriate support. Patients may indicate in a variety of ways that they want to talk to us about their illness, treatment or other problems. Of course, we too, consciously or unconsciously, give cues to patients and relatives about our own readiness to listen. We may sometimes recognise signs in ourselves which indicate whether or not we are ready to enter into discussion with a patient. It is easy to forget that uniforms and hospitals can be intimidating and patients and relatives often rely on us to indicate that we have set time aside to talk to them.

It has been recognised that non-verbal communication carries four times the weight of verbal communication (Henley 1973). Argyle (1992) claimed that: 'Non-verbal communication is a powerful indication of what we think and feel'. He also claims that it is more powerful than verbal communication. Stewart (1992) claims that words only constitute 10% of communication with tone constituting 40% and the remaining 50% being visual.

Benjamin (1981) emphasised the importance of congruence between verbal and non-verbal communication in effective counselling, and the importance of increasing our awareness of our non-verbal communications. He spoke of the insights gained through the use of video during counselling training sessions. Patients were aware of verbal and non-verbal aspects of communication. We communicate our support to others both verbally and non-verbally, and there must be consistency between these two forms of communication if we are to be perceived as genuine. In Bailey and Wilkinson's (1998) study, patients said that the good communicator must possess good non-verbal skills such as eye contact.

Perry (1996) studied exemplary oncology nurses and found non-verbal communication to be very important. Silence emerged repeatedly as an approach that was used by exemplary nurses in the study. Silence was important for listening and hearing the message. The second non-verbal theme identified by Perry was touch. Sometimes eye contact was combined with touch to provide a potent communication medium. Perry's third theme encompassing verbal and non-verbal behaviour was the use of humour. This was described as a lighthearted attitude among skilled nurses in the study. These nurses deliberately chose most of the time to see the positive and humorous side of situations to the benefit both of themselves and the patients. Benjamin (1981) also advocates the use of humour as a means of support. He points out that he does not mean ridicule or cynicism but a light touch of humour which stems from empathic listening and which reflects a positive outlook on life.

Below is a summary of the important elements of non-verbal communication:

- eye contact
- silence
- touch
- humour (verbal and non-verbal).

Non-verbal communication can convey to patients and relatives an impression of 'busyness' or 'availability'. It is important to make relatives feel at home and to minimise the institutional character of the establishment. My own research (Lugton 1987), showed that a personal approach by nurses to patients and relatives is appreciated, as shown in the statements below:

'I like how you feel at ease. Everybody is friendly.'

First impressions are important.

'My wife was naturally apprehensive but she came and

immediately had a sense of well being. I had maybe a five minute wait in reception and a comforting cup of tea that's obviously always given. Then I went into the ward and spoke to my wife and she was equally well comforted. When I looked at her bed and saw the flowers and the card with her name written on it and knowing that the emergency call had only gone to her doctor an hour before, I thought it was wonderful.'

Informality: breaking down barriers

Bailey and Wilkinson (1998) found in their study that the ability to foster a relaxed atmosphere emerged as the most important personal attribute documented by patients. Other attributes were:

- being approachable
- being friendly
- being calm
- being honest
- being sympathetic
- being non-judgemental
- having a sense of humour.

Patients and relatives appreciate an informal, friendly atmosphere and facilities which enable them to feel relaxed. In St Columba's Hospice there is a room where light refreshments are available and this is important for relatives who are visiting for most of the day. There is also a rest room where relatives can stay overnight, talk to the doctor in privacy, or simply be together as a family. Such simple, practical facilities are becoming more available in general hospitals and can do much to promote a feeling of welcome to relatives who are tired and under stress but who wish to remain close to their loved ones. A relative comments:

'It's such a relaxed atmosphere. It's easy to visit. It's small and people have got time.'

Use of first names

In my hospice research (Lugton 1987), several relatives commented on the way that nurses called patients by their first names and how this helped them to relax. People are, of course, asked about their wishes in this matter when they are admitted and their preferences are respected. There is often reciprocal use of first names between nurses and patients so putting the relationship on an equal basis and avoiding 'parent–child' overtones. This can be an integral part of the personal approach by nurses to patients and relatives, as Examples 7.1 to 7.3 show.

Example 7.1

'The staff are all so friendly. It's important to talk and feel that you're friends rather than nurse and patient. It's like a family for my wife and myself who have got no children, it's really a family.'

Example 7.2

'They had "Bob" on a little sign above his bed. It's a tiny thing, but again it gives you some feeling of warmth in the place rather than just the surname. Little things like that helped.'

Example 7.3

'The first names helped a lot. For the nurses, my father was "David" from the first moment he came in and several of the nurses knew my mother's name, Peggy. She liked that. She felt it was friendly.'

Like their relatives, many patients are apprehensive about admission to the hospice since it indicates that they are entering the final stages of their illness. Once they have overcome their initial anxieties about admission, however, most patients seem to be able to relax a little and their most common comment is satisfaction with the individual care and attention they receive. Patients often say that they feel safe in the hospice and their reassurance seems to derive from the perceived availability of staff and their ability to relieve distressing symptoms.

Availability, consistency and counselling skills

In a study of the Macmillan Nursing Service in West Lothian, Rutherford and McCleod (1986) stress the importance of availability, consistency and personal counselling skills in the relationships of Macmillan nurses to the patient and relatives at home. Relatives had found such support more helpful than practical advice, although the latter was also appreciated.

Availability

The availability of home care sisters is also appreciated in a hospice. It encourages a feeling in relatives and patients that expert help is always at hand, the sister being someone whom they know well, who is aware of their situation and who can be called upon when needed. Availability seems to be more important than frequent visiting, although the latter is appreciated. One relative felt able to cope as long as there was someone to turn to when things became too difficult at home:

'I had Dr Douglas and Sister Mary. They listened to me. They gave me the feeling, "When you can't manage, let

us know and we'll be there". I'd always the feeling that someone's there and you can say, "Look, I've come to the end now".'

The emotional rather than the physical strain of caring for the dying person at home is sometimes commented upon by relatives:

'The home care service helped mentally and in contact with the family. It was reassuring for my sister and I to know that someone was there to call on if things got too much. I think mentally, rather than physically, was the way the home care nurses helped. We felt somebody was taking an interest in us. They went out of their way to phone you and let you know what was happening. It made you feel safer.'

Relatives feel they can contact the home care team whenever they are in difficulties without their anxieties appearing trivial. This gives them extra confidence in caring for the dying person at home and often extends the duration of home care.

'You're all alone and you can't really phone up the GP. You don't want to get embarrassed by asking silly questions. It was nice when Mary, the home care sister, came down because we could speak to her. She was like part of the family, just coming in and knowing everybody that was there. She was easy to speak to. I had a better idea of what was going on. I thought that was good and I think it helped Mum too.'

The quality of the relationship that patients and relatives have with home care sisters is often commented upon. They are described as being 'relaxed', 'easy to speak to', 'supportive' and 'friendly'.

In the hospice as well, relatives mention the availability of nursing staff to talk to them as being very important. Relatives feel that the nurses try to get to know them when they come to visit (Examples 7.4 to 7.6).

> **Example 7.4**
>
> 'They seem to know you here, although it's only the third time I've been. First of all, there's more nurses here, but it's the same ones you see when you come in.'

It is important for nurses and doctors to take the initiative in communicating with patients and relatives.

> **Example 7.5**
>
> 'I've spoken to the sisters two or three times. I've spoken to one of the doctors and one or two of the nurses. The nurses sometimes come across and sit beside us when we're with father.'

> **Example 7.6**
>
> 'Before I used to be frightened to talk to anyone like a doctor. I feel that here you can relax and I'm not a relaxing person. The whole staff is so relaxed. I spoke to Dr Brown yesterday and he wasn't in a hurry to get away.'

Relatives are helped if they feel that nurses know them as a family and are aware of their circumstances, as Examples 7.7 and 7.8 show. One woman who had recently been bereaved describes the attitude of the nurses towards her parents.

> **Example 7.7**
>
> 'The staff were so kind. Mother was quite touched that the nurse who was with father at the end was quite upset with her. I think people were prepared to talk. The male nurse spoke to her for quite a while one night.'

A young man was concerned because his mother was asking to go home, a situation he could not cope with because he and his wife had had a baby daughter ten days previously. He particularly appreciated the doctor taking the initiative in approaching him to discuss the problem.

> **Example 7.8**
>
> 'One of the doctors came over and asked if she could see me for ten minutes. She said it wasn't the hospice that had suggested that Mum went home. She said they would only send her home if she was well enough to go. When she was in the hospital, the hospital was quite free with the information but you had to ask the right questions and you got the answers. I certainly appreciated being put in the picture and she did say if I had any concern to call into her office in passing or phone in.'

Telephone communication

The ready availability of information and support by telephone can greatly alleviate relatives' anxieties. We should encourage relatives to telephone as often as they wish for an update on a patient's condition, or to get details of their daily activities and general well being as this increases their sense of security. In a busy general hospital, it is helpful to staff if one relative maintains the telephone contact and relays the information to other family members. However, this may not be possible when a patient has a large family and many friends or when communication within the family is poor. We should ask relatives, on admission, whom we should contact if there is any deterioration in the patient's condition. If the next of kin is an elderly person or in poor health, a son or daughter may wish to be telephoned first in order to break the news of the decline more gently to a parent. It is useful to keep a daily record of each patient's activities and any fluctuations in mood as part of the documentation for the nursing care plan. Relatives appreciate information about whether the patient is eating their meals, sleeping well, or getting up in the mornings. Relatives often mention the helpfulness of telephone communication as shown in Examples 7.9 and 7.10.

Example 7.9

'I usually phone before I go to bed at night and I phone in the morning. It's very comforting to feel he's all right.'

Example 7.10

'I phoned last night and this morning and this afternoon. Everyone has been very helpful.'

Consistency

One or two nurses should try to develop a deeper relationship with each patient and his or her relatives so that they are given an opportunity to discuss any anxieties with someone known and trusted. If relationships are built up gradually in this way, patients and relatives feel more able to confide more fully their feelings and anxieties. If too many nurses are involved in care, patients and relatives may only be able to relate to them in a fairly superficial way. In the community, both patients and relatives like having the same nurse to visit, as they feel that she is interested in how they are coping with the situation, as well as in monitoring the patient's progress. Consistency is more difficult to achieve in a hospital or hospice setting where a number of nurses and other professionals are involved in care over a 24-hour period.

Counselling skills

The support of patients and relatives requires both sensitivity and counselling skills if it is to be effective. An essential element of counselling is that people are helped to adopt personal methods of coping with new experiences. For example, although many people experience the emotional reactions to loss described by Kubler Ross (1970), patients and relatives will respond with their own styles of coping. These will be influenced by their own personality, previous experiences with illness and loss, and their experiences of relationships with family and with health professionals. As nurses, we need to be skilled at helping patients and relatives to explore their feelings and anxieties and to identify their main concerns from among the many debilitating fears associated with terminal illness. One man particularly feared the effects on his wife of secondaries from a lung cancer:

'The doctor told me how her trouble is working and so forth. He said they would do their best to make it peaceful for her. He told us how the tumour will affect *her and how he thinks it should go, and he told us about the stages towards the end. I felt better after he had talked to me.'*

The ventilation of emotions is an important need of dying people and their relatives. There is a corresponding need for support from both nurses and other family members. Patients and relatives need opportunities to express their feelings and talk about family problems and other difficulties they are experiencing (*see* Chapter 5). In our relationships with patients and relatives, we should help people to identify their strengths and the family, professional, and other resources available to them in coping with their situation. For example, dying people and their relatives may need help in coping with extreme anxiety and fear of the future. Some relatives have a great fear of being unable to cope with the patient's terminal illness and with their own future during bereavement.

As nurses we should consider our willingness to respond in a personal as well as a professional way to the challenges and difficulties presented by families when a loved one is dying.

I have described the relationships with nurses that dying people and their relatives seem to find most supportive. The most valued features are availability, consistency and a counselling approach to support. Availability entails more than physical presence. It means having a familiar person to turn to in any kind of difficulty, great or small. Telephone support can greatly increase the availability of professional help. If one or two nurses take responsibility for supporting each dying person and his or her relatives, this allows for continuity and consistency of dialogue and for a deeper relationship to develop in which there is opportunity to confide in someone known and trusted. Such a 'covenant' relationship between the dying person and his or her carers goes beyond the normal contractual relationship between counsellor and client or professional and patient. It entails a willingness to listen and befriend without imposing duties on the patient. However, counselling skills are vital so that people can be helped to adopt personal methods of coping with their situations and so that nurses can respond to each person's needs on an individual basis.

Questions and exercises

1 In what ways do you make yourself more approachable/ available to communicate with dying people and their relatives (a) in the community or (b) in hospital? What do you do well? How could you improve what you do?
2 How could you minimise the 'institutional' character of a hospital ward and enable dying people and their relatives to feel more 'at home'?
3 In what ways could you improve 'consistency' or 'continuity' in relationships with dying people and their families?
4 To what extent would you describe your relationship with dying people as a 'covenant' relationship? Is that an honest assessment?
5 How positive and encouraging is your non-verbal communication? Study a video of yourself or ask a friend to comment on your non-verbal communication, noting such factors as eye contact, smiling, body position, and use of silence.

8

Potential communication problems

Getting close to terminally ill people can be emotionally draining for their carers, although, in my own experience, forming supportive relationships with distressed relatives can be even more demanding. The temptation is to protect ourselves from 'overinvolvement' by using distancing behaviour, such as talking to colleagues instead of to patients or unconsciously controlling communication with patients and relatives, so that people have little opportunity to express their real fears or negative feelings, such as anger or depression.

In palliative care, it is particularly important that stress experienced by patients and relatives should not be increased by poor communications, yet research has revealed, and our own personal and professional experience confirms, that great improvements are needed before patients and relatives receive the support which they have a right to expect from us.

Poor communication in palliative care

Communication problems have been highlighted as a source of increasing patient dissatisfaction with healthcare in the UK (Audit Commission 1993, National Cancer Alliance 1996). Patients interviewed by the National Cancer Alliance often felt that they had important information to pass on to health professionals involved in their care. Patients disliked being viewed as a hospital 'number' or 'tumour' to be processed, and stressed that they wanted to be treated with dignity and their personal needs respected. Wilkinson (1991) noted that nurses' communication skills did not appear to have improved over the last 20 years.

Psychological and psychiatric morbidity have been linked to situations in which patients' concerns remained undisclosed and unresolved (Parle *et al.* 1996). Some of the reasons for this apparent difficulty in supporting the terminally ill and their relatives will now be considered.

Negative professional attitudes to palliative care

An awareness of our own attitudes to death and bereavement, acceptance of our vulnerability and need for personal support will help us to approach dying patients and their relatives in a spirit of willingness to listen. We can offer support when asked, and admit that we do not have all the answers to their problems.

Wilkinson (1991) found that nurses used a variety of 'blocking' techniques such as changing the subject to prevent patients from speaking about their problems. This led to a poor assessment of psychological needs.

Inadequate assessment of patients' and carers' needs

Assessment acts as a basis for planning care on an individualised basis. However, Bailey and Wilkinson (1998) point out that health professionals find it difficult to actively enquire about patients' concerns and feelings. Booth *et al.* (1996) suggest that nurses are more comfortable dealing with patients' physical needs rather than addressing their emotional concerns and anxieties.

Lack of information from professionals to patients and relatives

Regrettably, several studies have confirmed that patients' and relatives' experiences of poor communication and support are widespread. Addington-Hall *et al.* (1991) found that 37% of relatives felt dissatisfied with the information provided by hospital personnel and by the way in which it was given. Carers wanted more information about the patient's condition and felt that they had not been warned that death was imminent. If family members do not know what to expect, they cannot use their time to the best advantage (Rose 1998). In my own hospice research, some relatives expressed considerable anger at what they perceived to be inadequate communication from doctors or nurses, as shown in Example 8.1.

> **Example 8.1**
>
> 'My father was in several hospitals and we met a lot of people. I had little faith in the ones I spoke to. I'd speak to different people and get different responses. They were overworked and understaffed. I wanted somebody to sit down and talk to me and I wanted one person that I felt I could trust.'

The development of counselling as a recognised professional specialty has shown that, although communication skills can be innate and that some people are naturally good communicators, new skills can also be learned and existing ones improved upon.

Doctor/nurse-centred approach or patient-centred approach?

The Nuffield Provincial Hospitals Trust Working Party (1978) reviewed extensive research on communications within the NHS and found evidence of poor medical interviewing and a lack of communication skills. In particular, they criticised the use of strings of routine questions which inhibited communication and the use of leading or closed questions which did not encourage patients to talk about their experiences of illness.

Numerous guidelines on communication with terminally ill patients have been produced. However, such guidelines may encourage professionals to give information routinely without exploring patients' understanding, concerns and desire for information (Maguire 1999). In my research with women having treatment for breast cancer, medical staff encouraged patients' involvement in treatment decisions (Lugton 1994). However, many patients were reluctant to take responsibility for decisions that might influence their prognosis, preferring to defer to medical opinion or make joint decisions with the doctors. In contrast, Alison, a finance consultant, wanted as much information about her treatment as possible:

'The doctor was always condemning me because I was asking her for the statistics. She said that most people can't cope with that. I said, "I would rather know". The doctor gave me some papers she'd written to read. The hormone therapy has failed. I was well prepared for the chemotherapy not to work. Twelve weeks chemotherapy *and the tumour went back to its original size. I didn't want to go through more chemotherapy. The surgeon spoke to me for a quarter of an hour and convinced me that I should go through with it.'*

The need for a patient-centred approach is obviously relevant to nursing as well as to medicine. The importance of allowing the patient or the relative to lead communication exchanges cannot be overemphasised. Only then will they be able to express their concerns when they wish to do so and ask for information and support when they perceive that they need it (Example 8.2). The question then changes from 'What to tell?' and 'When to tell?' to 'What does the patient want to know?' and 'At what pace can he or she cope with the knowledge?'.

Example 8.2

'I've been kept in the dark. I made a fool of myself saying, "There's no cancer" and there is. I'm really disillusioned. I'm very, very hurt.'

Some of the reasons for this apparent difficulty in supporting the terminally ill and their relatives will now be considered.

Time: quality and quantity in communications

Adequacy of communications is not only influenced by the time or numbers of staff available, but also, as has been indicated, by nurses' attitudes and communication skills. Quality is more important than quantity. In Hockley's (1983) study, time for nurses to get involved with patients and their families was often curtailed by lack of continuity of care due to the rapid changeover of medical and nursing staff. There is a need for nurses to make an assessment of patients' physical, psychological and social needs and the needs of their relatives for support. It is unlikely that all these needs will be met in a single interview at the time of admission or on the initial referral to the community nurse. A supportive relationship between nurse and relatives will not be developed when contacts are fleeting, hurried, or subject to interruption. My own experience has shown that a comparatively short time set aside to talk to patients and relatives and to listen to their concerns is greatly appreciated. There may be moments when a patient or relative feels particularly vulnerable and needs to express anxieties and fears. Experienced nurses will be aware that such moments often seem to occur when, for instance, the patient is having a bath or other intimate procedure carried out and when defences are lowered. These opportunities to share deep feelings should always be encouraged by nurses since, if they are ignored, they may not recur.

Interprofessional communication

Interprofessional communication can improve or hinder the psychological support which can be given to patients and relatives by the caring team. The Calman and Hine report (1995) states the importance of communication between primary care and specialist services, recommending that communication should be appropriate in time and content. Sofaer (1983) showed the importance of mutual communication between doctors and nurses in achieving pain control in surgical wards. Community nurses will recognise the importance of good communication between themselves and the hospital when a patient is discharged home. Unfortunately, the accompanying letter often details the diagnosis and treatment given but gives no indication of what the patient and relatives have been told about the illness or prognosis. In giving ongoing emotional support to patient and family and responding to their day-to-day needs, good communication between doctors, nurses and other professionals is essential as is the recognition that each profession has an important contribution to make. Frequent team meetings should be held to discuss the needs of dying patients and their families. In Hockley's (1983) study, it was noted:

> '*Some of the senior nurses in particular were very well motivated to try to incorporate principles of hospice care into the acute medical situations .... Often though, because of pressure of work and inexperience of symptom control, they lacked the necessary confidence when confronted with medical personnel.*'

Nurses too readily accept that the prime responsibility for achieving good symptom control is medical. However, confrontational methods of communication between nurses and doctors are not helpful in resolving problems for the patient's benefit. For example, nurses should accept responsibility in reporting a patient's pain and in monitoring the effects of analgesics. The patient's assessment of pain control using a pain chart may be more objective, detailed and less opinionated than the nurse's 'view' on the patient's drug regime. A nurse prepared to listen to patients and report their questions and anxieties, helps to avoid an unnatural distinction between 'telling' and 'not telling' patients about their condition.

Communicating with 'difficult' patients and relatives

Nurses may find certain patients 'difficult' to relate to for a variety of reasons. Stockwell's (1984) study of the unpopular patient found that nurses spent less time communicating with such people because they were demanding of their time and unrewarding as they were unappreciative of what was done for them. Dying people may try to cope with their anxieties and fears by being demanding or clinging, by complaining or sometimes by developing obsessional habits like keeping a note of all the medicines they receive and of the progress of their symptoms.

Some patients and relatives may become very withdrawn and uncommunicative. One such patient at St Columba's Hospice, a young man, was greatly helped by a nurse who sat on his bed and talked to him whenever she had the opportunity. Although he only replied in monosyllables at first, he gradually became more responsive.

Initiating communication

Some patients and relatives are reserved about approaching staff and speaking to them, especially when they are perceived as being very busy. It can be difficult, even in a relaxed atmosphere, for them to take the initiative in approaching staff. Patients and relatives may also be confused about nurses' uniforms and unsure of whom best to approach. Examples 8.3 to 8.6 from my own research (Lugton 1987) illustrate some of these difficulties from the relatives' viewpoint.

Example 8.3

'I've spoken to the nurses if they've been at the bedside or on the verandah. I've not really approached them to be quite honest. I leave it to them.'

Example 8.4

'I haven't spoken to anyone yet. I'm a bit shy.'

Example 8.5

'I haven't spoken to the doctor on his own yet. It's difficult when my husband's there. He would want to know what we were talking about.'

One relative requested that the nurses take more initiative in communicating.

Example 8.6

'I think it's important that someone speaks to the relative every other day or something like that.'

Relatives may sometimes be neglected, even when communication with the patient is good. Relatives may not be present when the doctor speaks to the patient, so a situation may easily arise where a person has been in hospital or a hospice for several days before the relative has spoken to a member of staff.

At the hospice, there is a system of 'starring' a patient's name when his condition has deteriorated or when the nurse or doctor wants to speak to the relatives. The receptionist then ensures that they do not leave before seeing the doctor or nurse.

Obtaining the required support

People communicate their deeper anxieties and fears in the context of a relationship of trust. It was this personal support which patients and relatives found so helpful with the home care service. One relative commented:

> *'At the moment, there are so many nurses I haven't figured them all out. I found the home care ones were very helpful. If I was really upset, I would go to Sister Sheila (home care). I've had that connection with her.'*

A few relatives felt that the nurses were friendly and approachable. However, these relatives needed support at a deeper level. Examples 8.7 to 8.10 reveal relatives' desire for more support and information from nursing staff. Again their perceptions of the staff's 'busyness' seem to deter relatives from approaching nurses.

Example 8.7

'I've only chatted to the nurses, sort of informal pleasantries and so on.'

Example 8.8

'I recognise the nurses and speak to them in passing but they're a bit busy when I'm there; they seem busy.'

Example 8.9

'I just don't know anything. I know they can't put a time on it. I'm supposed to be going on holiday in a fortnight's time. I decided not to go. I just asked sister if the doctor had spoken to her and what he said. You don't want to be bothering them. They're busy and they've got a lot to do.'

Example 8.10

'I haven't had any discussions with the nursing staff. If I've any criticisms it's that. If someone after two days said, "Oh Mrs Y, can we see you for a few minutes", but nobody in fact has. Nobody actually stopped me and said "You know, we are doing X, Y, Z". That might have been helpful.'

Communicating spiritual needs

Walter (1997) describes three models of spiritual care evident in hospices. The first focuses on religious rites and preparing people for heaven. The second is founded on compassion and practical care for the dying. The third is focused on the search for meaning. This latter view is also shared by Holst (1994) and Simmonds (1994) who stress the need to work alongside people in their search for meaning. Burnard (1987) defines spiritual distress as the inability to invest life with a meaning.

Most nurses will remember moments when medical solutions seemed inadequate to meet a distressing situation, and when a very ill patient or anxious relative seemed to be asking for something to give meaning to their suffering or to the prospect of a premature death. Perhaps we have felt embarrassed or inadequate in such a situation or when asked about our own beliefs. Spiritual care is now considered to be part of the total care of our patients and the spiritual dimension to caring also extends to support of relatives and friends. To what extent then, should we, as nurses, consider spiritual care to be part of our work? Spirituality has become less visible in our healthcare institutions and has increasingly come to be considered a very personal and private matter. People's spiritual needs are not always very apparent and can be overlooked because of the intensity of medical and nursing care. We may be uncertain of being drawn into conversation about spiritual matters. Maybe we should be more willing to examine our attitudes towards spiritual care as we do our styles of communication with patients or our attitudes towards death and dying.

For those who have a strong personal faith, pastoral care may seem a natural part of their nursing role. Those who do not have strong religious convictions may feel that they have little to offer the patient in this area. Some nurses may feel that any attempt at pastoral care by nurses is an intrusion into a patient's privacy or into the role of the clergy. There are obvious dangers in an evangelical approach to people who are terminally ill. The patient must always take the lead in asking questions. However, for spiritual care to be helpful, it has to be seen as available to those who may be seeking it. A delicate balance must be maintained between any attempt to force religious views on vulnerable patients and creating an atmosphere in which patients are allowed their right to seek spiritual comfort and to express their spirituality in their own way. For example, creating a quiet and private environment for prayer or reception of the sacraments can add immeasurably to the dignity of such occasions. Although spiritual and emotional care are closely linked, pastoral care is not concerned primarily with expertise in communications and counselling or knowledge of theology but with being a companion on life's journey (Campbell 1981). Spiritual pain is not alleviated if attention is paid only to people's physical needs, however good the standard of care. Spiritual distress arises whenever the individual is unable to answer the questions:

- Who am I?
- Why is this happening?
- What is the meaning of life?
- What is the meaning of suffering and death?
- What have I done to deserve this?
- Am I being punished?
- Do I really matter?

In my experience, spiritual questions raised by patients have related to broken relationships, fears about death and dying, fears of a judgemental God, and regrets about the past. Frankl (1987) emphasises the importance of finding meaning in life, saying:

> 'A man who has the "why" to live can put up with almost any "how".'

Non-verbal communications are important when a patient may be unable to express his thoughts or needs in words.

A primary goal of spiritual care is to help individuals to achieve peace of mind. The key to pastoral care is availability, being ready at any time and in any way to respond to the needs of the patient. Anyone who is trying to give spiritual help cannot hide behind his or her professional status but has to sometimes acknowledge his or her own weakness and inability to provide all the answers to difficult questions. The offer to pray with, or on behalf of, someone who cannot pray due to weakness or tiredness can be greatly appreciated. However, there is no need to be concerned with finding the right words to meet every situation as long as genuine concern is evident in every aspect of care. We should not feel hesitant about trying to give spiritual help and sharing patients' own beliefs if we feel that the patient is asking and such a sharing would be appropriate. Those who feel unable to respond on a personal level can work with their colleagues or with the clergy for the benefit of the patient. It is important that staff do not have 'no go areas' so far as communication is concerned.

An interdenominational working party at Sir Michael Sobell House (1991) discussed the medical and nursing aspects of spiritual care. It stressed the importance of the carer 'being there' without feeling guilty or embarrassed, listening, and sometimes allowing the patient to express anger.

I have outlined some familiar communication problems in palliative care. When such difficulties arise, solutions may depend on asking ourselves the right questions. For example, communication is a dialogue, hence the need to be aware of what patients and relatives want to know, as well as being concerned with how and what we should tell them. Some difficulties in communication may be more apparent to the staff than perceived by patients and relatives. For example, a heavy workload may mean that less time can be spent with patients and relatives than we would wish. However, mean-ingful and effective communications need not necessarily be lengthy. Indeed, some of us who have been on the receiving end of long-winded monologues in which we found it diffi-cult to state our own views, would readily recognise that brevity can be a virtue! So long as we give equal priority to communication as we do to other aspects of care and realise that support can be planned and evaluated, we will not go far wrong. Interprofessional communication takes place against a background of mutual role expectations, but such expectations can be changed and become more realistic if the professionals involved are more prepared to be open with each other and show greater understanding of each other's responsibilities.

Questions and exercises

1 How do you try to communicate with a terminally ill person who seems anxious, withdrawn or depressed? Are you usually successful? If not, why not?

2 Think back to the last time you had difficulties communicating with a dying person. What did you see as the problem areas for (a) him or her and (b) for you? What did you do well? In retrospect, how could you have been more supportive?

3 What do you feel is your role, if any, in talking to dying people or their relatives about spiritual matters?

4 Recall an instance where a patient appeared to be in spiritual distress. What were the verbal and non-verbal cues? How did you respond?

5 How do you ensure that your support is patient- or relative-centred and not nurse-centred? Record a conversation with a patient. Do you explore patients' understanding, concerns and desire for information before giving information and support? How many times do you or the patient lead the conversation?

9

A three-stage model of support

Friendliness and warmth from professional staff are clearly appreciated by patients and relatives, but sometimes a deeper level of support is indicated. People under stress value having a sympathetic listener. Many also seek someone who will help them to clarify what they should do to cope more effectively with the difficulties brought about by serious illness. To be effective, the support of terminally ill people and their relatives requires an individual approach from nursing staff combined with counselling skills.

Assessment and support must be ongoing to be effective. Maslow (1962) has described an ascending order of human needs from basic physical and security needs to needs for giving and receiving love and for self-development. These needs are just as much present in dying people as in those who have a long span of life ahead. A small, unpublished study by Nimmo (1982) has reinforced an impression that, though patients may present largely physical problems on admission, emotional, social and spiritual concerns emerge as important at later interviews. It may be that professional staff make priorities out of problems which they can solve therapeutically. In nursing, there has been an emphasis on the active work of giving physical care rather than on the equally demanding work of communicating with and giving support to patients and their families. Patients and their relatives and professional carers may perceive different priorities of care, hence the need for continuing support, so that all the concerns of patients and relatives are allowed to emerge. Ramirez (1999) maintained that the need for support among people with cancer might be at one of three levels. These were as follows:

- Level 1 – Everyone needs effective, supportive, communication.
- Level 2 – One in four need supportive counselling.
- Level 3 – One in ten need specialist intervention such as cognitive therapy.

These levels of need by patients mirror the three levels of competence in palliative nursing advocated by Webber (1993). Support for the patient's identity or self-concept is necessary at every level of communication so that the person retains a core sense of self and control of self which is undamaged by the illness or fears of the future (Lugton 1994).

The Egan model of counselling

Counselling differs from other forms of 'helping' relationships in assisting people to help themselves by becoming aware of available choices, making their own decisions, or coming to terms with a new experience. Egan (1990) developed a skills model of counselling, which, like the nursing process, has three stages. In the exploration stage the person is helped to assess their own situation and needs. This may take some time. A picture of patients' and relatives' needs can be built up over a number of interactions with the nurse, and any problems or anxieties they want to explore can be identified. In the understanding stage, the person is helped to reach a new understanding of their situation and to clarify what they might do to cope effectively. The third stage is helping the person to implement decisions and plans and consider possible consequences. A care plan for the patient and relatives is made out. The nurse, as counsellor, can use his or her skill and experience to be aware that the person is ready to move from one stage to another, thus ensuring that they go at the person's pace and not their own. When giving support, it is important to remember how easy it is for professionals to make such vulnerable people dependent upon them, and thereby to increase their sense of helplessness. Nurses can create difficulties for themselves by asking questions such as, 'What should the patient be told about his illness?' instead of, 'What does the patient want to know about his illness?'. Support of patient and family should always be preceded by careful assessment of their expressed needs. This allows an individual and flexible approach to be adopted for each person. Heron (1990) recognised the need in counselling to balance authoritative interventions, such as advice and information giving and confrontation, with facilitative interventions, which are cathartic, catalytic and supportive. This means that power can be shared more equally between professional and client.

The Egan model of counselling and support and its application to terminal care will now be examined in more detail. An outline of the model is shown in Box 9.1.

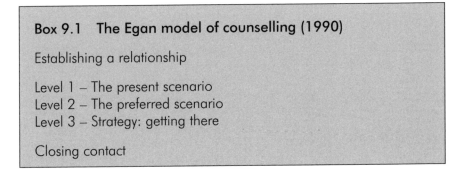

Box 9.1   The Egan model of counselling (1990)

Establishing a relationship

Level 1 – The present scenario
Level 2 – The preferred scenario
Level 3 – Strategy: getting there

Closing contact

Establishing a relationship with patient and family

The first contact between nurse, patient and relative(s) will have an important influence on later relationships. Time, availability and privacy are important in establishing good relationships. In hospital, it is preferable if one or two nurses can take responsibility for the support of a particular patient and family to ensure continuity of dialogue and to build up a trusting relationship. Information important to the care of the patient and family can be shared with members of the professional team. The nurse responsible for the care of a particular patient and family should take the initiative in sustaining contact with them, so letting them know that she has set time aside for any concerns they may want to discuss.

Timing of support sessions

Timing is important in establishing any relationship. Relatives and patients are often under stress at the time of admission to hospital, or on an initial home visit. They may be anxious about the suspected diagnosis or about signs of recurrence of an earlier disease. The hospital environment can be stressful in itself, presenting new and sometimes unpleasant experiences and a bewildering number of faces to be remembered. Any session at this initial stage should be as brief as possible to minimise stress. A further session (or sessions) is, nevertheless, needed to explore patients' and relatives' needs and to plan emotional support. As the aim of the sessions is to allow dying people and their relatives to explore areas of concern to them, it should be made clear from the outset that there is no set agenda for discussion nor any information which must be obtained. If family communications seem to be blocked in any way, it may be helpful to talk to the patient and family together.

Hospital–community liaison

There may be considerable information available about the social circumstances of patients referred from the community to hospital or vice versa. Some of this information may be invaluable in planning the giving of effective support, and good hospital–community liaison is important. For example, a note should be made of patients' and relatives' awareness of diagnosis, if appropriate. A family tree may be useful in identifying those relatives and friends of the patient who may need support. A visit by the community nurse to the hospital could provide hospital nurses with information about a patient's home circumstances, or help to prepare for discharge.

Level 1: Identifying and clarifying problem situations

The first stage in developing supportive relationships would be an exploration of patients' and relatives' needs and anxieties conducted in an atmosphere where privacy and freedom from interruption are guaranteed. Patients need to tell their stories and discuss their problems. Some will find this easy to do, while others will find it more difficult. Nurses need skills to enable patients to tell their stories and to provide support for them while they do so. The skills demanded of the interviewer at this stage are as follows:

1 active listening/attending
2 clarifying the main concerns/challenging faulty interpretations
3 responding to feelings.

Active listening/attending

By giving total attention to what the other person is saying about their experiences and feelings, the helper can create a climate of empathy and trust. Patients or relatives should be encouraged to talk freely. They may want to talk about a problem that is worrying them or just express their feelings to a sympathetic listener. It is important to give people the chance to do this rather than to subject them initially to a multitude of questions. When not pressurised to respond to the nurse's agenda they will be more likely to present a fuller version of their various problems. Egan (1990) notes that there are three levels of attending to clients; the microskills level, the body language level and the presence level. The microskills, which indicate attending, can be summarised by the acronym SOLER. These are as follows:

- S – face the client squarely, turning towards him or her
- O – adopt an open posture, with arms and legs uncrossed
- L – lean towards the other person
- E – maintain fairly steady eye contact
- R – be relaxed.

Awareness of non-verbal communication through the body, for example, tensions and facial expressions, is very important. Finally, verbal and non-verbal behaviour should send the same message of total attention of the nurse to the patient and of their commitment to his or her welfare.

Clarifying the main concerns/challenging faulty interpretations

Patients and relatives may respond to an invitation to talk by describing many anxieties or problems. It is important to find out which of these are the main concerns. Open questions

encourage the person to develop an open and 'giving' conversation and explore thoughts and feelings, rather than giving
brief, defensive responses. Gradually, as the session progresses, the helper can begin assisting the person to focus on
the most important areas of concern (for the person, not the
helper). For example, if relatives are anxious about coping at
home, they could be asked to give examples of situations
where they feel anxious. The nurse could challenge relatives'
feelings that they are not coping with caring for the patient at
home by helping to make relatives more aware of the good
care they are already giving. New understanding may help
people to see blind spots or patterns in their behaviour of
which they were previously unaware. For example, a female
relative who has been curt and irritable with nursing staff
may be helped by making her realise that she is angry with
them for 'taking over' the care of her loved one, which is
making her feel inadequate and guilty. With new understanding, she begins to realise that she has often responded to
serious events in her life by taking control, and that this has
often antagonised people. As the main concerns emerge, these
can be explored in more depth in stage two of the interview.

Responding to feelings

Both patients and relatives experience emotions associated
with grief, for example, denial, anxiety, anger and guilt.
They want the opportunity to express their feelings and to
talk about the difficulties they are experiencing. Strong negative feelings which are not expressed can make coping with
terminal illness significantly more difficult for patients and
relatives. As nurses, we can help the person explore these
often painful emotions by sensitive listening and reflecting of
feelings. The person gets the chance to 'ventilate' feelings,
which, in itself, can bring a sense of relief, and also the
person becomes more aware of the reasons behind these feel-

ings. We can help them find signs of hope in complex situations.

Level 2: Developing a preferred scenario

At this stage, we can help the person to become as clear as possible about their concerns and what they might do to cope with them more effectively. We can help them to develop a picture of the problem situation as it would be if improvements were made. We can help them to set outcome priorities. The skills demanded of the helper are as follows:

1 responding and leading/exploring possibilities
2 promoting understanding/developing agendas
3 information giving
4 giving advice.

Responding and leading/exploring possibilities

We can direct the person's attention to areas that seem important to them. In this way, they can be helped to develop a range of more hopeful alternatives to their problem situation.

Promoting understanding/developing agendas

The helper encourages the person to gain insight into their feelings and circumstances. As the dialogue progresses and mutual confidence and trust grow, it is easier to ask more sensitive questions. Patients can be helped to make choices. Relatives of a dying person might be asked 'Have you thought at all about the future?'. Many relatives are willing to talk about this and some will speak of tentative plans they are making. Egan (1990) calls this 'translating preferred scenario possibilities into viable agendas'.

Information giving

Patients and relatives need information from staff at different stages of the illness and at a level with which they can cope. Information should only be given after assessing the patients' and relatives' desire for it. For example, some relatives do not want to know the patient's prognosis and many do not want detailed information about the terminal illness itself, symptoms or treatment. Relatives do, however, need frequent updating on the person's condition to allay their anxiety.

Giving advice

Advice should be given with caution, only when requested and when the patient's and relatives' situation has been explored. Relatives may ask for advice because they want a professional assessment of the situation and feel incompetent to make it themselves. There are dangers in giving specific advice when, for example, the patient's condition is uncertain. People who appear extremely ill may sometimes improve and live for several weeks or months. Other people may deteriorate suddenly and die just at the moment when the relative had decided to go home to rest.

Level 3: Making plans

Stage three of the interview involves identifying possible actions and their respective implications for support by professionals. Fairly immediate action is sometimes indicated and the help of the nursing staff may be required. For example, there may be problems of communication in some families or parents may be concerned about what to tell the children about the terminal illness. The skills required of the helper at this stage are as follows:

1 choosing the best strategies
2 planning action
3 anticipating situations.

Choosing the best strategies

Patients and relatives are encouraged to choose the strategies that best fit their needs, preferences and resources.

Planning action

Patients and relatives are encouraged to formulate a plan to alleviate any problems, to attain important goals and improve their quality of life. Staff may be able to help in this. For example, a patient may wish to make out a will to ensure adequate provision for his or her family, or relatives may wish to plan a special celebration for the patient's birthday or for a wedding anniversary.

Anticipating situations

In some areas, patients or relatives may not be in a position to make definite decisions or plans. Some relatives have to experience bereavement before they know how they will cope with, for example, role changes or moving house. Nevertheless, they will be in a better position to make wise decisions, having had the opportunity to discuss their situation, consider alternatives and clarify their feelings beforehand.

Closing contact

The supportive relationship between a nurse and a terminally ill person has a natural end when the person dies. In the support of bereaved relatives, however, there is not always an obvious time to begin closing contact. There are certain points to be considered which may prompt closing contact.

- The person may have needs which the helper cannot meet. For example, there may be signs of abnormal grieving, such as severe depression or an inability to make a beginning to life without the deceased person.
- The person may need referral to another agency or professional in order to receive appropriate help. For example, the bereaved person may need medical or psychiatric help.
- If the helper is no longer able to continue to support the person, perhaps because of professional commitments, referral to another agency for further support might be appropriate. For example, a health visitor or district nurse might refer a bereaved person to a group such as CRUSE where both individual counselling and group support are available. Such a referral would, of course, only be made with the bereaved person's consent.
- Contact may be closed when the aims of the supportive relationship seem to have been met. Sometimes this may be done gradually, with visits from the helper becoming less frequent as the person seems to be progressively more able to cope alone.

It may be difficult to close contact with a person whom we, as nurses, have grown to like and who is grateful for the care received from us. However, it is important to allow the person to grow in independence, and it is necessary for our own emotional well being that we do not see ourselves as the only ones capable of giving such support. We also have obligations to other patients and relatives who may have a more pressing need for our help. The ability to close a supportive relationship successfully at the appropriate time is, therefore, as important as its establishment. The memory of both first and last impressions will probably remain with relatives for the rest of their lives.

An example of how the counselling model could be applied to the support of dying people and their relatives was given earlier, when a relative was described as being angry with the nurses for 'taking over' the care of her loved one. She can be helped to explore and gain insight into her feelings. In the action stage of the counselling session she may decide that she needs to express more often how anxious, worried and lost she feels over her loved one's imminent death. She may identify a close friend who she thinks she can trust to confide in, and she may decide to tell her how she feels the next time they meet. The counselling nurse can explain how she can become more involved in the nursing of her husband, if she wishes, and that she can telephone the hospital whenever she feels anxious or wishes to be updated on his condition.

Areas to be explored with dying people and their relatives

The preceding chapters have indicated the areas of likely concern to dying people and their relatives, and which concerns the nursing staff should explore with them. These concerns are now identified below.

Awareness of diagnosis: patients and relatives

Patients' and relatives' awareness of the terminal diagnosis should be noted. Any communication between patients, relatives and staff about the diagnosis or prognosis should be recorded so that the various professionals involved in the patient's care can give continuity of emotional support.

Coping with terminal illness: patients and relatives

Nurses should note how patients and relatives are coping with the terminal illness, since awareness does not always indicate acceptance. The principal carer should be identified, as the burden of care, both physical and emotional, may have taken its toll. Negative feelings in both patient and relative should be explored so that they can be helped to cope with their situation in as positive a manner as possible.

Anxiety

Areas of anxiety should be explored with both patients and relatives so that opportunities to alleviate these fears are not lost.

Perceived support: patients and relatives

The extent of perceived support seems to be more important than the size of a person's social network in alleviating loneliness. Opening up communications within the family of a terminally ill person can increase the support members give to each other. Patients can often give great support to each other. Relatives who do not perceive themselves as being well supported seem to be more at risk of having a difficult bereavement. All these situations have implications for support from professional staff.

Planning action: the patient's priorities and plans

Stage three of the counselling process involves making plans, which have been mutually agreed between patient and professional carer. Seemingly unimportant things can make an enormous difference to the quality of life of terminally ill people. If the nurse is aware of a patient's priorities, they can help the patient to use their limited energies to maximum effect in the short time that may be left to them and create some happy memories for relatives. In cases where a very ill person has become withdrawn and uncommunicative with their family, relatives may need particular help and support so that they realise that this is not a rejection of them, but part of the illness.

Relatives' priorities and plans

When death has been anticipated for weeks or months, relatives have often begun to think of the future without the patient and some begin to make tentative plans. Where the terminal illness is at all protracted, relatives may have been obliged to adopt new roles and a new lifestyle. For example, they may be considering moving house. Loss of income may mean changes in lifestyle. When encouraging the relatives to think about and discuss their own needs, the nurse could discourage them from making overly hasty decisions based on their present feelings, which they may later regret.

The aim in this chapter has been to indicate the needs of dying people and their relatives for an appropriate level of support from nursing staff. Some difficulties which terminally ill people and their relatives experience have been discussed and the implications for psychological support considered. It is not intended that only the nurse should be seen as giving this help. The support of colleagues in the professional team is essential. In Chapter 2, the importance of team meetings and case conferences in promoting mutual respect and understanding among the various professionals was emphasised. Mutual respect and cooperation are necessary for any one team member to develop skills in counselling and support. The comments of colleagues from their own and other disciplines (and indeed from patients and relatives) can be invaluable in improving nurses' communication skills. A hierarchical approach to communication in terminal care with each member of a team taking his or her cue from the top of the professional hierarchy is unlikely to be helpful to patients and is stressful for the staff concerned.

Nurses should make a more effective contribution to the provision of support to dying patients and their relatives, and the multidisciplinary team should be constantly seeking to improve the level of its collective skills. If a team approach to the support of dying people and their relatives is accepted as necessary, there are obvious implications for nursing education, since nurses have a key role. The improvement of communication and counselling skills is now considered important for both student and registered nurses. More interdisciplinary counselling courses are needed to promote mutual awareness and understanding of roles among professionals.

A good team approach to care does not just happen. Its members have to work together and grow in mutual understanding, confidence and support. Usually a doctor is the team leader, but other members have important roles. A nurse may find that his or her role is that of coordinating the contributions of the various team members, for the benefit of the patient and family. For example, a district nurse will liaise with the GP, the Macmillan nurse, or the health visitor, and various agencies such as the home-help service or the night-sitter service, in providing care for the terminally ill person. Nurses' active role as advocate for the patient is vital. Since they are often in daily contact with the patient and family, they are also best placed to be aware of their expressed needs. Very often a nurse, both in the hospital and in the community, is the key person in communicating between the terminally ill person, their family and professional carers. Nurses should be encouraged to expand their already growing contribution to this essential area of patients' and relatives' care, whether in the community, hospital or hospice.

Questions and exercises

1 Which aspects of the Egan model of counselling might you find particularly helpful in improving your own communication in terminal care?
2 Think of a recent situation in which you supported a patient or relative. Did you enable him or her to move through all three stages of Egan's helping model? Were there any barriers within yourself or the patient/relative that prevented this happening?
3 When talking to dying patients and their relatives, how much time do you spend:
   • listening, responding, clarifying?
   • talking – leading?
   What does this say about you?
4 When talking to dying people and their relatives how much time do you spend:
   • giving them advice?
   • giving them information?
   • asking them about their feelings, anxieties, and problems?
   What does this say about you?
5 How do you help terminally ill people and relatives identify their priorities and make their own plans? What do you do well? How could you be more helpful to patients and relatives in this area?
6 Do you have any difficulties closing contact with bereaved relatives? In what ways could you make this easier?

Postscript

This postscript has been written by the daughter of a patient in St Columba's Hospice.

'This book has been written openly about caring for the terminally ill patient in hospices, hospitals and at home. It covers many aspects of the worries, fears and anxieties of patients and relatives. It discusses the relationship between staff and patients in St Columba's Hospice, Edinburgh and touches on subjects such as day visits, which familiarise the patient with the hospice. It speaks of the relative's role when a loved one is being cared for in the hospice and the need to be able to converse with staff at the hospice. Simply to talk or ask questions which may be worrying the relative can lend support when a doctor or nurse, with confidence and experience, can speak frankly about the patient's condition. It also deals with family support in the bereavement itself. At the hospice the "caring" for the patient and the "dignity" of the patient are factors which are highly important.

The home care service and the Macmillan nurses who play an important part in the hospice caring service, are also discussed in their role of visiting patients in their homes, dealing with their

*needs, and becoming familiar with relatives and home circum-
stances.*

*From my own personal experience this care was given to my own
family during my mother's illness and tremendous support was
received. Each visit from the nurse was on a friendly basis when
my mother and my family always felt at ease in discussing any
problems. Questions were always frankly and honestly answered.
There was always a feeling of "trust" and a knowledge that my
mother was in the hands of extremely qualified and sympathetic
people.'*

In my research (Lugton 1994), a patient with breast cancer
illustrated beautifully how good communication had built up
a strong, trusting relationship between herself and her health
visitor:

*'She (health visitor) is my lifeline. I know she's there. I
suppose it's a bit like a kid with a night light. You know
it's there if you want it. She really made a tremendous
difference.'*

A patient (1994)

Appendix: Useful addresses

Alzheimer's Disease Society
Gordon House,
10 Greencoat Place,
London SW1P 1PH.
Helpline: 0845 300 0336
Administration: 020 7306 0606

British Association for Cancer United Patients (BACUP)
3 Bath Place,
Rivington Street,
London EC2A 3DR.
Telephone: 020 7920 7206
Provides information for cancer patients and others; produces leaflets on various aspects of cancer; gives telephone support.

CARE (Cancer After-care and Rehabilitation Society)
Lodge Cottage,
Church Lane,
Timsbury,
Bath BA3 1LF.
Telephone: 0761 70731
Offers support and advice to cancer patients and their families, including information about hospices and welfare rights.

Compassionate Friends
53 North Street,
Bristol BS3 1EN.
Helpline: 0117 953 9639
Administration: 0117 966 5202
Offers support and help for people suffering the loss of a child; leaflets for parents, professionals, friends and relatives and a library.

Crossroads (Association of Crossroads Care Attendance Scheme)
10 Regent Place,
Rugby,
Warwickshire CV21 2PN.
Telephone: 01788 573653
Have schemes in various parts of the UK that allow families to have a break from caring at home for handicapped people.

CRUSE: National Organisation for the Widowed and their Children
Cruse House,
126 Sheen Road,
Richmond,
Surrey TW9 1UR.
Helpline: 0870 167 1677
Administration: 020 8939 9530
Counselling service with branches throughout UK; wide range of literature, bereavement counselling courses.

Foundation for the Study of Infant Death
(Cot Death Research and Support Associations)
Artillary House,
11–19 Artillary Row,
London SW1P.
Telephone: 020 7233 2090
Advice and counselling for newly bereaved parents. Sponsors research and produces useful leaflets.

Gay Switchboard
BM Switchboard
PO Box 7324,
London N1 9QS.
Telephone: 020 7837 7300
Twenty-four hour information and help service for lesbians and gay men; will also refer those recently bereaved to their bereavement project.

Institute of Family Therapy
24–32 Stephenson Way,
London NW1 2HX.
Telephone: 020 7391 9150
It provides high level family therapy training, short courses, workshops and family clinical services. Free counselling is available to newly bereaved families through the Elizabeth Raven Memorial Fund.

Jewish Bereavement Counselling Service
Coburn House,
Tavistock Square,
London WC1H 0EZ.
Telephone: 020 8349 0839
Will send trained volunteer counsellors to bereaved; operates in Greater London but can refer to other projects and individuals elsewhere.

Macmillan Cancer Relief
89 Albert Embankment,
London SE1 7UQ.
Telephone: 0945 601 6161
Support, advice and help concerning palliative care for people with cancer; provides short-stay homes and nursing services for patients; can provide financial help for those in need; apply through social worker, GP or social services.

Marie Curie Cancer Care
89 Albert Embankment,
London SE1 7TP.
Telephone: 020 7599 7729
Advisory and counselling service for cancer patients and relatives; can provide day and night nursing service for patients at home and runs welfare grant scheme.

Motor Neurone Disease Association
PO Box 246,
Northampton NN1 2PR.
Helpline: 08457 626262
Administration: 01604 250505
Gives advice and information for sufferers of this disease; grants for home nursing, hospice care and holidays; leaflets available.

Sargent Cancer Care for Children
Griffen House,
161 Hammersmith Road,
London W6 8SG.
Telephone: 020 8752 2800
Can provide cash grants to parents of children with cancer to help pay for clothing, equipment, etc. (Hospital social worker can supply application form.)

Scottish Cot Death Trust
Royal Hospital for Sick Children,
Yorkhill,
Glasgow G3 8SJ.
Telephone: 0141 357 3946
Advice and counselling for newly bereaved parents. Sponsors research and produces useful leaflets.

St Christopher's Hospice Information Service
51–59 Lawrie Park Road,
Sydenham,
London SE26 6DZ.
Telephone: 020 8778 9252
Can provide information about approximately 87 hospices in the UK.

Stillbirth and Neonatal Death Society (SANDS)
28 Portland Place,
London W1N 4DE.
Helpline: 020 7436 5881
Administration: 020 7436 7940
Offers advice and long-term support, via local groups, to newly bereaved parents of stillbirths and/or of babies who die in their first month of life.

Sue Ryder Foundation
Central Office,
2nd Floor,
114–118 Southampton Row,
London WC1B 5AA.
Telephone: 0787 280252
Runs 20 homes for the physically handicapped and for both terminal and convalescent cancer patients; can also provide domiciliary care teams.

Tenovus Cancer Information Service
11 Whitchurch Road,
Cardiff CF4 3JN.
Telephone: 029 2062 1433
Gives information on all types of cancer; can refer to appropriate organisations for further help; produces leaflets and educational material including films and video cassettes.

The Rainbow Trust
Claire House,
Bridge Street,
Leatherhead,
Surrey KT22 8BZ.
Telephone: 01372 363438
Aims to relieve pain and suffering among chronically or term-
inally ill children and their families and to advance the educa-
tion of the public in the care of sick children.

The Traumatic Stress Clinic
73 Charlotte Street,
London W1T 4PL.
Telephone: 020 7530 3666

Ulster Cancer Foundation (Cancer Information Service)
40–42 Eglantine Avenue,
Belfast BT9 6DX.
Telephone: 01232 663281
Supports and informs the public and health professionals in
all areas of concern related to cancer problems; operated by
experienced cancer nurses; literature available.

Winston's Wish
Gloucester Royal Hospital,
Great Western Road,
Gloucester GL1 3NN.
Winston's Wish provides a grief support programme for children who have experienced the death of a parent, brother or
sister. Gloucestershire-based, it is free to families who live in
that county. Places are available, at a charge, for families
living outside the county. Winston's Wish also has a National
Development Programme that provides training and advises
people wanting to set up similar services in their local
communities.

References

Adam J (2000) Discharge planning of terminally ill patients home from an acute hospital. *International Journal of Palliative Nursing* **6 (7)**: 338–45.

Addington-Hall JM, MacDonald LD, Anderson HR and Freeling P (1991) Dying from cancer, the views of bereaved family and friends about the experiences of terminally ill patients. *Palliative Medicine* **5**: 207–14.

Ad Hoc Committee on Medical Ethics (1984) 1: History of medical ethics, the physician and the patient, the physician's relationship to other physicians, the physician and society. *Annals of International Medicine* **101**: 129–37.

Ajeman I (1995) The interdisciplinary team. In: D Doyle and G Hanks (eds) *Oxford Textbook of Palliative Medicine*. Oxford University Press, Oxford, pp. 17–27.

Anderson J (1988a) Facing up to mastectomy. *Nursing Times* **84 (3)**: 36–9.

Anderson J (1988b) Coming to terms with mastectomy. *Nursing Times* **84 (4)**: 41–4.

Argyle M (1992) *The Psychology of Interpersonal Behaviour* (4e). Penguin, Harmondsworth.

Audit Commission (1993) *What Seems to be the Matter: communication between hospital and patients*. National Health Service Report No. 12. HMSO, London.

Bailey K and Wilkinson S (1998) Patients' views on nurses' communication skills: a pilot study. *International Journal of Palliative Nursing* **4 (6)**: 300–5.

Beaver K, Luker KA and Woods S (2000) Primary care services received during terminal illness. *International Journal of Palliative Nursing* **6 (5)**: 220–7.

Benjamin A (1981) *The Helping Interview* (3e). Houghton Mifflin, Boston.

Bihm E and Elliot I (1982) Conception of death in mentally retarded persons. *Journal of Psychology* **3**: 205–10.

Billings JA (1995) Palliative medicine update: depression. *Journal of Palliative Care* **11 (1)**: 48–54.

Booth K, Maguire P, Butterworth T and Hillier V (1996) Perceived professional support and the use of blocking behaviour by hospice nurses. *Journal of Advanced Nursing* **24**: 522–7.

Bowlby J (1981) *Loss, Sadness and Depression*. Penguin, Harmondsworth.

Brietbart W, Bruera E, Chochinov H and Lynch M (1995) Neuropsychiatric syndromes and psychological symptoms in patients with advanced cancer. *Journal of Pain and Symptom Management* **10 (2)**: 131–41.

Buckman R (1992) *How to Break Bad News*. Papermac, Basingstoke.

Buckman R (1995) *What You Really Need to Know About Cancer*. Macmillan, London.

Burnard P (1987) Spiritual distress and the nursing response; theoretical considerations and counselling skills. *Journal of Advanced Nursing* **12**: 377–82.

Calman K and Hine D (1995) *A Policy Framework for Commissioning Cancer Services*. DoH, London.

Campbell A (1981) *Rediscovering Pastoral Care*. Darton, Longman and Todd, London.

Carkuff RR (1969) *Helping and Human Relations: a primer for lay and professional helpers.* Holt, Rinehart and Winston, New York.

Cathcart F (1991) Bereavement and mental handicap. *Bereavement Care* **10**: 9–11.

Cathcart F (1994) *Understanding Death and Dying.* A series of three booklets for the client, relative and professional carer. Available from the British Institute of Learning Disabilities, Wolverhampton Road, Kidderminster DY10 3PP.

Cathcart F (1995) Death and people with learning disabilities: interventions to support clients and carers. *Journal of Clinical Psychology* **34**: 165–75.

Costello J (2000) Truth telling and the dying patient: a conspiracy of silence? *International Journal of Palliative Nursing* **6 (8)**: 398–405.

Davies B, Reimer JC and Maatens N (1994) Family functioning and its implications for palliative care. *Journal of Palliative Care* **10 (1)**: 29–36.

Dunne K and Sullivan K (2000) Family experiences of palliative care in an acute hospital setting. *International Journal of Palliative Nursing* **6 (4)**: 170–8.

Egan G (1990) *The Skilled Helper: a systematic approach to effective helping.* Brooks/Cole Publishing, California.

Fallowfield L (1995) Psychosocial interventions in cancer. *British Medical Journal* **311**: 1316–17.

Finnannon JL (1995) Analysis of psychiatric referrals and interventions in an oncology population. *Oncology Nursing Forum* **22 (1)**: 87–92.

Frankl V (1987) *Man's Search for Meaning.* Hodder and Stoughton, Sevenoaks.

Glaser BG and Strauss AL (1965) *Awareness of Dying.* Aldine Publishing Co., Chicago.

Hampe SO (1975) Needs of the grieving spouse in a hospital setting. *Nursing Research* **24 (2)**: 113–20.

Heaven C and Maguire P (1996) Training hospice nurses to elicit patient concerns. *Journal of Advanced Nursing* **23**: 280–6.

Henley N (1973) *Power, Sex and Non-verbal Communication*. Newbury House Rowley, Massachusetts.

Henley S (1983) Bereavement by suicide. *Bereavement Care* **2**. CRUSE, London.

Heron J (1990) *Helping the Client: a creative practical guide*. Sage Publications, London.

Herth K (1990) Fostering hope in terminally ill people. *Journal of Advanced Nursing* **15**: 1250–9.

Hockley J (1983) *An Investigation to Identify Symptoms of Distress in the Terminally Ill Patient in the General Medical Ward*. City and Hackney Health District, Nursing Research Paper 2.

Hockley J and Dunlop R (1990) *Terminal Care Support Teams*. Oxford Medical Publications, Oxford.

Holst LE (1994) The role of chaplains in the end of life decisions. *Hospital Health Network* **9**.

Jencks M (1995) *The Daily Telegraph*, July 20.

Jobling M (1975) *Bereavement in Childhood: a summary of research findings*. National Children's Bureau Information Service, London.

Johnson JL (1991) Learning to live again: the process of adjustment following a heart attack. In: JM Morse and JL Johnson (eds) *The Illness Experience*. Sage Publications, London.

Johnston G and Abraham C (2000) Managing awareness; negotiating and coping with a terminal prognosis. *International Journal of Palliative Nursing* **6 (10)**: 485–500.

Katz J and Sidell M (1994) *Easeful Death*. Hodder and Stoughton, London.

Kelly M (1991) Coping with an ileostomy. *Social Science and Medicine* **33**: 115–25.

Kindlen K and Walker S (1999) Non-specialist nurse education in palliative care. In: J Lugton and M Kindlen (eds) *Palliative Care: the nursing role*. Churchill Livingstone, Edinburgh.

Kreiger D (1982) *The Renaissance Nurse*. Harper and Row, New York.

Kristjanson L and Ashcroft T (1994) The family's cancer journey: a literature review. *Cancer Nursing* **17**: 1–17.

Kubler Ross E (1970) *On Death and Dying.* Tavistock Publications, London.

Levy LH, Derby JF and Martinoski KS (1992) The question of who participates in bereavement research and the bereavement risk index. *Omega: The Journal of Death and Dying* **25**: 225–38.

Lewis CS (1961) *A Grief Observed.* Faber and Faber, London.

Lindemann F (1944) Symptomatology and management of acute grief. *American Journal of Psychiatry* **101**: 141–9.

Lugton J (1987) *Communicating with Dying People and their Relatives.* Mosby, London.

Lugton J (1994) *The Meaning of Social Support: a descriptive study of informal networks and of health visitors' formal role in supporting the identity of women with breast cancer* (unpublished PhD). Nursing Studies Department, University of Edinburgh.

Lugton J (1997) The nature of social support as experienced by women treated for breast cancer. *Journal of Advanced Nursing* **25**: 1184–91.

Lugton J (1999) Support processes in palliative care. In: J Lugton and M Kindlen (eds) *Palliative Care: the nursing role.* Churchill Livingstone, Edinburgh, Chapter 4.

Lund DA, Caserta MS and Dimond M (1993) The course of spousal bereavement in later life. In: MS Stroebe, W Stroebe and RO Hansson (eds) *Handbook of Bereavement Theory, Research and Intervention.* Cambridge University Press, New York.

Lynam MJ (1990) Examining support in context, a redefinition from the cancer patient's perspective. *Sociology of Health and Illness* **12 (2)**: 169–94.

McIntosh J (1977) *Communication and Awareness in a Cancer Ward.* Croom Helm, London.

McIntyre R (1996) *Nursing support for relatives of dying cancer patients in hospital, improving standards by research* (unpublished PhD). Department of Nursing and Community Health, Glasgow Caledonian University, Glasgow.

McIntyre R (1999) Support for family and carers. In: J Lugton and M Kindlen (eds) *Palliative Care: the nursing role.* Churchill Livingstone, Edinburgh.

Maguire GP (1995) Psychosocial interventions to reduce affective disorders in cancer patients: research priorities. *Psycho-oncology* **4**: 113–9.

Maguire GP (1999) Improving communication with cancer patients. *European Journal of Cancer* **35 (10)**: 1415–22.

Maguire GP, Tait A, Brooke M *et al.* (1980) Effect of counselling on psychiatric morbidity associated with mastectomy. *BMJ* **281**: 1454–6.

Maslow A (1962) *Towards a Psychology of Being.* Van Nostrand Reinhold, New York.

Massie MJ, Gagnon P and Holland JC (1994) Depression and suicide in patients with cancer. *Journal of Pain and Symptom Management* **9 (5)**: 325–40.

Mills M, Davies HT and Macrae WA (1994) Care of dying patients in hospital. *BMJ* **309**: 583–5.

Murphy SA (1988) Mental distress and recovery in a high risk bereavement sample 3 years after untimely death. *Nursing Research* **37 (1)**: 30–5.

National Cancer Alliance (1996) *Patient-centred Cancer Services: what patients say.* National Cancer Alliance, Oxford.

Nimmo G (1982) *A study of the principal distresses experienced by patients with terminal cancer and the importance attached to them by patient and physician* (unpublished). St Columba's Hospice, Edinburgh.

Nuffield Provincial Hospitals Trust (1978) *Talking with Patients: a teaching approach.* Nuffield Provincial Hospitals Trust, London.

Øvretveit J (1995) Team decision making. *Journal of Interprofessional Care* **9 (1)**: 41–51.

Parkes CM and Weiss RS (1983) *Recovery from Bereavement.* Basic Books, New York.

Parle M, Jones B and Maguire P (1996) Maladaptive coping and affective disorder among cancer patients. *Psychological Medicine* **26 (4)**: 735–44.

Penson J (1990) *Bereavement: a guide for nurses.* Chapman and Hall, London.

Perry B (1996) Influence of nurse gender on the use of silence, touch and humour. *International Journal of Palliative Nursing* **2**: 7–14.

Plant R (1987) *Managing Change and Making it Stick.* Gower, Aldershot.

Ramirez A (1999) Proceedings of the British Psychosocial Oncology Society Conference, December, London.

Raphael B (1984) *The Anatomy of Bereavement. A Handbook for the Caring Professions.* Anchor Brendon, Essex.

Rose K (1998) Perceptions related to time in a qualitative study of informal carers of terminally ill patients. *Journal of Clinical Nursing* **7**: 343–50.

Rutherford M and McCleod C (1986) *The West Lothian Macmillan Service: the first three years.* Unpublished report.

Seale C (1991) Communication and awareness about death: a study of a random sample of dying people. *Social Science and Medicine* **32**: 943–52.

Seale C (1999) Awareness of method: re-reading Glaser and Strauss. *Mortality* **4 (2)**: 195–202.

Seo M, Tamura K, Hiroshi S *et al.* (2000) Telling the diagnosis to cancer patients in Japan: attitude and perception of patients, physicians and nurses. *Palliative Medicine* **14**: 105–10.

Sheldon F (1993) The needs to be met, 16–19. In: *Needs Assessment for Hospice and Specialist Palliative Care Services: from philosophy to contracts.* Occasional Paper 4, National Council for Hospice and Specialist Palliative Care Services, London.

Simmonds AL (1994) The chaplain as a spiritual and moral agent. *Humane Medicine* **10 (2)**: 103–7.

Skilbeck J, Mott L, Smith D *et al.* (1997) Nursing care for people dying from chronic obstructive airways disease. *International Journal of Palliative Nursing* **3 (2)**: 100–6.

Slevin ML, Stubbs L, Plant HJ *et al.* (1990) Attitudes to chemotherapy: comparing the views of patients with cancer with those of doctors, nurses and general public. *BMJ* **300**: 1458–60.

Smith S (1996) A study to investigate (a) patients' recollections of their encounters with doctors during their cancer care and (b) the number of doctors encountered during this period. In: *Progress in Palliative Care: Conference Report.* Scottish Partnership Agency for Palliative and Cancer Care, Edinburgh.

Sobell Publications (1991) *Mud and Stars: The Impact of Hospice Experience on the Church's Ministry of Healing.* Sobell Publications, Oxford.

Sofaer B (1983) Pain relief – the importance of communication. *Nursing Times*, December 7.

Stedeford A (1981) Couples facing death: psychosocial aspects. *BMJ* **283**: 1033–6.

Stewart W (1992) *The A–Z of Counselling: theory and practice.* Chapman and Hall, London.

Stockwell F (1984) *The Unpopular Patient.* Croom Helm, London.

Strachan JG (1981) Reactions to bereavement: a study of a group of adult mentally handicapped hospital residents. *Journal of the British Institute of Mental Handicap* **9 (1)**: 20–1.

Stroebe M, Gergen M, Gergen K and Stroebe W (1993a) Broken hearts of broken bonds. *American Psychologist* **47**: 1205–12.

Stroebe MS, Stroebe W and Hansson RO (eds) (1993b) Bereavement research and theory: an introduction to the handbook. In: *Handbook of Bereavement Theory, Research and Intervention.* Cambridge University Press, New York.

Tait A (1988) Whole or partial breast loss, the threat to womanhood. In: M Salter (ed) *Altered Body Image, the Nurse's Role.* John Wiley, Chichester, pp. 167–77.

Thompson IE, Melia KM and Boyd KM (1983) *Nursing Ethics*. Churchill Livingstone, Edinburgh.

Twycross RG (1995) *Symptom Management in Advanced Cancer*. Radcliffe Medical Press, Oxford.

Wakefield A (2000) Nurses' responses to death and dying: a need for relentless self care. *International Journal of Palliative Nursing* **6 (5)**: 245–51.

Walshe C (1997) Whom to help? An exploration of the assessment of grief. *International Journal of Palliative Nursing* **3 (3)**: 132–7.

Walter T (1994) *Revival of Death*. Routledge, London.

Walter T (1996) A new model of grief and bereavement and biography. *Mortality* **1 (1)**: 7–25.

Walter T (1997) The ideology and organisation of spiritual care: three approaches. *Palliative Medicine* **11**: 21–30.

Webber J (1993) *The Evolving Role of the Macmillan Nurse*. Macmillan Cancer Relief, London.

Wilkinson S (1991) Factors which influence how nurses communicate with cancer patients. *Journal of Advanced Nursing* **16**: 677–88.

Wilkinson S, Roberts A and Aldridge J (1998) Nurse–patient communication in palliative care; an evaluation of a communication skills programme. *Palliative Medicine* **12**: 13–22.

Wilson CM (1985) *Stress in Hospital Nursing*. The Division of Clinical Psychology Newsletter, No. 48, British Psychological Society.

Winnicot D (1965) *The Maturational Processes and the Facilitating Environment*. Hogarth Press, London.

Woodhall C (1986) A family concern. *Nursing Times and Nursing Mirror* **82**: 31–3.

Worden W (1991) *Grief Counselling and Grief Therapy: a handbook for the mental health practitioner* (2e). Routledge, London.

Wright B (1996) *Sudden Death: a research base for practice* (2e). Churchill Livingstone, Edinburgh.

Wright K and Dyck S (1984) Expressed concerns of adult

cancer patients' family members. *Cancer Nursing* **37**: 1–374.

Zimmerman L, Story KT, Gaston-Story F and Rowles JR (1996) Psychological variables and cancer pain. *Cancer Nursing* **19 (1)**: 44–53.

Further reading

Backhurst D (1992) Debate – on lying and deceiving. *Journal of Medical Ethics* **18**: 63–6.

Bascom PB (1997) A hospital based comfort care team: consultation for the seriously ill and dying patients. *American Journal of Hospice and Palliative Care* **14 (2)**: 57–61.

Dunlop RJ and Hockley JM (1998) *Hospital Based Palliative Care Teams: the hospital–hospice interface.* Oxford University Press, Oxford.

Ellershaw JE, Peat SJ and Boys LC (1995) Assessing the effectiveness of hospital palliative care teams. *Palliative Medicine* **9**: 145–52.

Herth K (1993) Hope in the family caregivers of terminally ill people. *Journal of Advanced Nursing* **18**: 538–48.

Horn S and Munafo M (1997) *Pain: theory, research and intervention.* Open University Press, Buckingham.

Lugton J (1997) Health visitor support for patients with breast cancer – 1. *Nursing Standard* **11 (33)**: 33–7.

Lugton J (1997) Health visitor support for patients with breast cancer – 2. *Nursing Standard* **11 (35)**: 35–8.

Pearce C and Lugton J (1997) Holistic assessment of patients' and relatives' needs. In: J Lugton and M Kindlen (eds) *Palliative Care: the nursing role*. Churchill Livingstone, Edinburgh.

Russell G (1993) The role of denial in clinical practice. *Journal of Advanced Nursing* **18**: 938–40.

Twycross RG (1993) Symptom control, the problem areas. *Palliative Medicine* **7 (Supplement 1)**: 1–8.

Index